中华传统经典养生术

（汉英对照）

(Chinese- English) Traditional and Classical Chinese Health Cultivation

Chief Producer　Li Jie	总策划　李　洁
Chief Compilers　Li Jie　Xu Feng　Xiao Bin　Zhao Xiaoting	总主编　李　洁　许　峰　肖　斌　赵晓霆
Chief Translator　Han Chouping	总主译　韩丑萍
English Language Reviewer　Lawrence Lau	英译主审　劳伦斯·刘

古音六字诀

Gu Yin Liu Zi Jue (Six Healing Sounds)

编著　孙　磊
Compiler　Sun Lei

翻译　韩丑萍
Translator　Han Chouping

上海科学技术出版社
Shanghai Scientific & Technical Publishers

I0103947

图书在版编目（CIP）数据

古音六字诀：汉英对照/孙磊编著；韩丑萍译.
—上海：上海科学技术出版社，2015.5
（中华传统经典养生术）
ISBN 978-7-5478-2550-1

Ⅰ.①古…　Ⅱ.①孙…　②韩…　Ⅲ.①气功-健身运
动-汉、英　Ⅳ.①R214

中国版本图书馆CIP数据核字（2015）第042360号

古音六字诀

编著　孙　磊

上海世纪出版股份有限公司
上海科学技术出版社　出版

中国图书进出口上海公司　发行

2015年5月第1版
ISBN 978-7-5478-2550-1/R·872

Gu Yin Liu Zi Jue (Six Healing Sounds) · 古 音 六 字 诀

顾问委员会
Advisory Committee Members

主任

徐建光　陈凯先　严世芸　郑　锦

Directors

Xu Jianguang　Chen Kaixian　Yan Shiyun　Zheng Jin

副主任

施建蓉　　胡鸿毅　季　光　张怀琼　余小明　劳力行

Vice Directors

Shi Jianrong　Hu Hongyi　Ji Guang　Zhang Huaiqiong
Yu Xiaoming　Lao Lixing

学术顾问

严世芸　林中鹏　林　欣　李　鼎　俞尔科　王庆其
潘华信　潘华敏　姚玮莉　赵致平　李　磊

Academic Advisers

Yan Shiyun　　Lin Zhongpeng　Shin Lin　　Li Ding　　Yu Erke
Wang Qingqi　Pan Huaxin　　Pan Huamin　Yao Weili
Zhao Zhiping　Li Lei

编纂委员会

Compilation Committee Members

总策划

李　洁

Chief Producer

Li Jie

总主编

李　洁　许　峰　肖　斌　赵晓霆

Chief Compilers

Li Jie　Xu Feng　Xiao Bin　Zhao Xiaoting

副总主编

孙　磊　陈昌乐　倪青根

Vice Chief Compilers

Sun Lei　Chen Changle　Ni Qinggen

总主译

韩丑萍

Chief Translator

Han Chouping

副主译

赵海磊

Vice Chief Translator

Zhao Hailei

Gu Yin Liu Zi Jue (Six Healing Sounds) · 古音六字诀 · 2 · 编纂委员会 · Compilation Committee Members

中文主审
周敦华　李小青

Chinese Language Reviewers
Zhou Dunhua　Li Xiaoqing

英译主审
劳伦斯·刘

English Language Reviewer
Lawrence Lau

编　　委（按姓氏笔画排序）

叶阳舸	许　峰	孙　磊	李　洁	李小青	肖　斌
吴璐一	沈晓东	陆　颖	陈　驰	陈昌乐	周敦华
赵　丹	赵晓霆	赵海磊	倪青根	韩丑萍	

Editorial Board Members (listing names in alphabetic order)

Ye Yangge	Xu Feng	Sun Lei	Li Jie
Li Xiaoqing	Xiao Bin	Wu Luyi	Shen Xiaodong
Lu Ying	Chen Chi	Chen Changle	Zhou Dunhua
Zhao Dan	Zhao Xiaoting	Zhao Hailei	Ni Qinggen
Han Chouping			

项目资助

Acknowledgement

· 上海市新闻出版专项扶持资金项目

· 上海市中医药三年行动计划（2015—2018年）"基于〈中华气功史陈列馆〉科普教育基地为核心的〈中医气功文化平台〉建设"（项目编号：ZY3–WHJS–1–1010）

· Shanghai Press and Publication of special support funds program

· The Three-Year Action Plan for Chinese Medicine in Shanghai (2015–2018) on Construction of Qigong Cultural Platform in the Museum of Chinese Qigong History (Program No: ZY3–WHJS–1–1010)

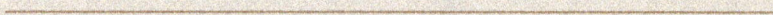

序

Foreword

欣闻上海市气功研究所编写的《中华传统经典养生术》丛书即将出版,这是中华原创医学文明传播的一件盛事,特致贺忱。

中华传统养生术源远流长,其中导引术更是重要的组成部分,它先于针、灸、药、医而形成,是中华民族最早用以防治疾病、养生保健的重要方法之一。现存早期文献《庄子》《吕氏春秋》《黄帝内经》以及考古发现《引书》《导引图》中均有关于养生导引及其具体方法的记载。此后绵绵数千年的历史长河中,中华养生导引术不断丰富、发展与创新,在自我实践中形成千门万法,在去伪存真中完善理论体系。20世纪后叶,古之导引术又以现代"气功"的面目再次席卷中华大地,并享誉海内外。时至今天,中华导引术仍然以其"人天合一"的整体观思想与丰富多姿的养生导引方法独立于世界自然医药之林,滋润着人类身心世界。事实表明,中华导引术已经形成为一门博大精深的学术体系。它所研究的是人之物质基础(精)与自组织能力(神)相互关系的规律,是关于"人"——这个地球上最复杂系统达到和谐与协调的一门学问。

我和上海市气功研究所相识逾30年,该所自20世纪70年代的中医研究所开始,气功与导引就是关注、研究的重点领域;80年代中期更名气功研究所后,更是全力着眼于现代气功的研究与中华导引术的弘扬。《中华传统经典养生术》是上海市气功研究所多年来所教授养生导引术、气功功法的汇编与总结,对于帮助学习、普及推广现代导引术具有较好的价值。希望此丛书的出版,能够进一步带动当前养生导引术在海内外的健康发展,推动中华优秀文化走向世界各地。

是以为序。

林中鹏

2015年3月

It is with great pleasure that I learn the *Traditional and Classical Chinese Health Cultivation* series compiled by the Shanghai Qigong Research Institute will be published soon. This means a lot to the spread of Chinese medical civilization.

Traditional Chinese health cultivation has a long-standing and well-established history. As an important part of health cultivation practice, Dao Yin exercise was used for disease prevention and treatment as well as life cultivation before acupuncture, moxibustion and herbal medicine. The recordings of *Dao Yin* and its specific exercise methods can be traced back to the *Zhuangzi, Lü Shi Chun Qiu* (The Annals of Lü Buwei), *Huang Di Nei Jing* (the Yellow Emperor's Inner Classic) and archaeologically unearthed books such as *Yin Shu* (a book on Dao Yin) and *Dao Yin Tu* (Dao Yin Diagram). After this, the thousands of years have witnessed the enrichment, progress and innovation of Chinese *Dao Yin* practice, coupled with emergence of numerous methods and perfection of its theoretical system. In late 20th century, the ancient *Dao Yin* exercise became exceptionally popular across China in the form of 'qigong'. Today, Chinese *Dao Yin* exercise remains flourish with its holistic 'Man-Nature Unity' idea and various exercise methods that benefit both body and mind. Facts show that there is a profound academic system behind Chinese *Dao Yin* exercise. This system studies the interactions between material foundation (essence) and self-organization ability (mind). In other words, it studies the way to achieve harmony and coordination of human being—the most complex system on earth.

I've established a friendship with the Shanghai Qigong Research Institute for 30 years. Ever since its founding in 1970s as a Research Institute of Chinese Medicine, qigong and *Dao Yin* have always been the research priorities of the Institute. The focuses on qigong and *Dao Yin* have been more highlighted in 1980s when the Institute was renamed as a Qigong Research Institute. I firmly believe that the

Traditional and Classical Chinese Health Cultivation series are of great significance in popularizing modern *Dao Yin* exercise. I sincerely wish the book series can further promote *Dao Yin* exercise at home and abroad and spread excellent Chinese culture.

For this, I wrote this forward.

Lin Zhongpeng
March 2015

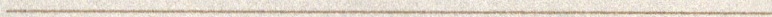

前　言

气 以 臻 道

　　农历乙未早春，正是上海市气功研究所创建三十周年之际，恰逢气功学术发展枯木迎春之季。在此，我们谨向海内外气功学界发出倡言——构建现代气功"气以臻道"的学术思想。

　　所谓"气以臻道"，首先是指气功学术发展必须树立一个大方向，即中华传统文化精神的最高目标——"道"；其次是指通过对"气"的感性体验与理性认知，使生命更趋向"道"，与"道"合一。道者，规律、目标也；气者，方法、途径也；臻者，趋向、完善也。气-道共同构成"气以臻道"学术思想内核。其中气为实、主行，是具体之指；道为虚、主理，是抽象之喻。气因道而展，道由气而实；气以道归，道以气显；气借道而实际指归，道假气而理性论证。气功学术发展必须气、道并重，互印互证，理行一贯。两者既各尽其责、各擅其能，又有主从之别。"道"因标指形上本体而为万法归宗之源；"气"每描述形下万法而成法法生灭之流。"道"经思维抽象提炼，揭示规律、规则之理性思辨；"气"常直叙主观感觉，表述体会、觉受的感性认识。道-气，一主一从，一虚一实，构成中华气功学术思想的本质内涵。

　　"气以臻道"学术思想之主体是"道"，是指向真理之道路，是学术文化人文精神的体现，也是先人用身心去实践生命运化规律的心得体验，古人称为"内证之学"。"道"的外延旁及"功"和"术"，可以包括各种神秘现象、气功现象、特异现象，古人称为"神通法术"。当今，现代科学研究介入传统气功学术是时代进步的表现，它为我们观察生命奥秘打开了一个全新的视角。透过唯象的研究，重新激发起人类对生命的思考与敬重，重新挖掘出科技文明下的人文精神，而非单纯地将生命物质化，这才是现代科学介入传统气功的人文价值所在。

有鉴于此，我们倡议构建现代气功研究之"气以臻道"学术思想，让中华传统文化与现代科学携起手来，揭示生命真谛，回归大道本源。

上海市气功研究所

2015年春

Advocacy for *Qi-Dao Harmony* in Modern Qigong Practice

The year 2015 is a Chinese new year of yin wood sheep (*Yi Wei* in Chinese). Wood, in Chinese culture on five elements (*Wu Xing*), is connected to the season of spring. The year 2015 also marks the 30th anniversary of the founding of Shanghai Qigong Research Institute. With a strong belief that the spring of 2015 will bring new hope to qigong study, we hereby advocate the concept of 'Qi-*Dao Harmony*' for its academic advance.

The term *Qi-Dao Harmony* has two underlying implications. First, it implies that *dao* is the ultimate goal of traditional Chinese culture and the general orientation for academic qigong advance. Second, it implies that our lives shall combine into one with the *dao* through perception and understanding of qi. In summary, this term means to achieve and perfect *dao* through qi exercise. The 'qi' here is weighted and refers to practice. The '*dao*' here is unweighted and refers to principles. Without *dao*, qi cannot extend; without qi, *dao* cannot become weighted. Qi finds its origin in *dao* and *dao* manifests itself in qi. Qi returns to *dao* eventually and *dao* supports qi theoretically. It's essential for people in academic qigong field to pay equal attention to qi and *dao*. The two have a principal-subordinate relationship. The metaphysical *dao* is the origin of all methods. The physical qi is the practice of all methods. *Dao* is about the abstract thinking and reveals the laws and rules. Qi is about the subjective feelings and tells experience and perception. Qi and *dao* constitute the essence of academic idea in Chinese qigong.

Let's get a deeper look into the concept of *Qi-Dao Harmony*. Also known as the 'learning of internal evidence', *dao* is the way to truth. It contains humanistic spirit and physical and mental experience of our ancestors. *Dao* extends to exercise (*gong*) and a variety of magic arts including mysterious, qigong and extrasensory phenomena. Today, modern scientific qigong research offers a new insight into the mysteries of life. The phenomenological research rekindles our reflection and respect towards life and enables us to re-discover humanism from modern civilization greatly impacted by science and technology. This is the real value of scientific research on traditional qigong in this materialized world.

To this end, we advocate the academic concept of '*Qi-Dao Harmony*' in modern qigong research. We believe the combination of traditional Chinese culture and modern science can help us to reveal the truth of life and return to the origin of the great *dao*.

Shanghai Qigong Research Institute
Spring 2015

编写说明

Words from the Compilers

中华传统养生术根植于中国传统哲学、中医学和养生学，是人体自我身心锻炼的有效方法。

随着倡导"主动健康"概念日益深入人心，具有调身、调息、调心功能的中华传统养生术，以其传统的养修理论、独特的身心效果蜚声海内外，引起世人的广泛关注。但近期国内外少见中国传统养生术的书籍出版，尤其没有成套、成系列的经典养生类作品问世，更缺乏英汉对照的专业著作。

上海中医药大学上海市气功研究所研究人员在前期研究工作基础上，精选中华传统经典养生术共八种，从历史源流、功法理论、特色要领、图解动作、分解说明与具体运用几方面进行中文编纂，由上海中医药大学中医英语专业人员进行翻译。并邀请专家进行中文审稿，邀请美国友三中医药大学Lawrence Lau先生审定英文翻译。

本套丛书详细地将八种中华经典养生术以图文并茂、视频摄像的形式记录下来，配以光盘，非常方便学习与传播，尤其便于海外养生爱好者以英语来学习。

本套丛书编纂过程中，得到上海市中医药三年行动计划（2015—2018年）"基于〈中华气功史陈列馆〉科普教育基地为核心的〈中医气功文化平台〉建设"（项目编号：ZY3-WHJS-1-1010）资助。

编者

Traditional Chinese health cultivation includes a variety of body-mind exercises, which are deeply rooted in ancient Chinese philosophy and medicine.

Today, the concept of 'health initiative (an ability to achieve physical, mental and social well-being)' has become well recognized.

Traditional Chinese health cultivation exercises are attracting worldwide attention because of their unique effects in regulating the breathing, body and mind. However, there are few books in this regard, especially the classical book series. There are even fewer bilingual Chinese-English versions of these books.

Based on their previous studies, research staff at the Shanghai Qigong Research Institute compiled eight traditional and classical health cultivation exercise methods, covering their history, theoretical foundation, characteristics and key principles, illustrated movements and application. Then these contents have been translated by professional interpreters at Shanghai University of Traditional Chinese Medicine. The Chinese version was reviewed by an expert team. The English version was reviewed by Dr. Lawrence Lau at the Yo San University of Traditional Chinese Medicine.

In addition to illustrations and videos are also available for readers, especially overseas health cultivation fans to learn.

This books series have been funded by the Three-Year Action Plan for Chinese Medicine in Shanghai (2015–2018) on Construction of Qigong Cultural Platform in the Museum of Chinese Qigong History (Program No: ZY3–WHJS–1–1010).

Compilers

目 录

Table of Contents

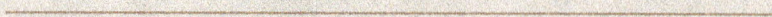

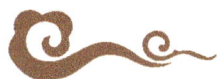

古 音 六 字 诀 • *Gu Yin Liu Zi Jue* (Six Healing Sounds)

History

源流

六字诀，又称"六气诀""六气法"，属于吐纳之法。六字诀历史悠久，历代版本较多，根据其操作姿势分类主要有吐纳六字诀、导引六字诀、静功六字诀三大类。古音六字诀是导引动作结合六字诀的一种导引六字诀，发音以吴音为基础，导引动作以明代流行的延年六字总诀为基础，故又称"吴音延年六字诀"。

Liu Zi Jue, also known as *Liu Qi Jue* or *Liu Qi Fa*, is one of the common forms of breathing exercise. Styles of *Liu Zi Jue* vary in different generations. In terms of exercise posture, there are three major categories — *Tu Na* (exhalation and inhalation) *Liu Zi Jue, Dao Yin* (guiding and stretching) *Liu Zi Jue* and *Jing Gong* (static exercise) *Liu Zi Jue.* As a subtype of *Dao Yin Liu Zi Jue, Gu Yin Liu Zi Jue* is based on the Wu (including southern part of Jiangsu Province, northern part of Zhejiang Province and eastern part of Anhui Province) dialect and *Yan Nian* (prolonging life) *Liu Zi Jue* in the Ming Dynasty (1368–1644). Consequently, it's also called *Wu Yin Yan Nian Liu Zi Jue.*

远在春秋战国时期，《老子》有"或嘘或吹"之说，西汉河上公注："嘘，温也。吹，寒也。"《庄子·刻意》篇中说："吹呴呼吸，吐故纳新，熊经鸟申，为寿而已矣。"由东汉时期张道陵（俗称张天师）作序，阴长生真人所撰的《太清金液神丹经》已有六字诀的记载。

The recording of *Liu Zi Jue* can be traced back to the Spring-Autumn and Warring-State Period (770 BC–476 BC). The *Laozi* States, '... one can aspirate the syllabus of *Xu* or *Chui*'. According to the Heshang gong[1] commentary in the Western Han dynasty (202 BC–9 AD), '*Xu* removes pathogenic warmth and *Chui* removes pathogenic cold'. The outer chapter 8 of *Zhuang Zi* records, 'Breath in and out in various manners, exhale the old and inhale the new, walk like a bear and stretch their neck like a bird to achieve longevity'. The detailed description of *Liu Zi Jue* was recorded in the *Tai Qing Jin Ye Shen Dan Jing* (Great Clarity: Scripture on the Divine Elixirs of Golden Liquid) written by Yin Chang Sheng Zhenren (literally means a true man) and foreworded by Zhang Dao-ling[2] in the Eastern Han dynasty (25 AD–220 AD).

目前普遍认为六字诀的正式记载见于南朝齐梁时期的道教茅山派代表人物之一的陶弘景所著的《养性延命录》一书。陶弘景（456—536年），南朝齐梁间道士、医学家，丹阳秣陵（今江苏南京）人，在医药、炼丹、天文历算、地理、兵学、铸剑、经学、文学艺术、道教仪典等方面都有深入的研究。他自幼聪慧，约10岁时即读葛洪《神仙传》，深受影响。陶弘景36岁时梁朝取代齐朝而立，辞官拜陆修静弟子孙游岳为师，成为上清派传人，隐居句曲山（茅山）华阳洞，并遍历诸有名大山，访求仙药。当时，他深受梁武帝萧衍的信任，梁武帝多次赠官不受，但梁武帝有关国家大事都要向他咨询，所以时人对他有"山中宰相"的称号。

It's now generally believed that *Liu Zi Jue* was officially recorded in the *Yang Xing Yan Ming Lu* (Records on Nourishing Character & Prolonging Life) by Tao Hong-jing (456–536), a leading figure of the Maoshan School of Taoism who lived in the

---

1. The name Heshang Gong means an old man who dwells by the side of the river, and some have identified the river in question to be the Yellow River. As the legend goes, he was an expert on the Laozi and famous for his commentary on *Dao De Jing*.
2. Also known as Zhang Tianshi (Celestial Master Zhang), an Eastern Han Dynasty Taoist figure credited with founding the Way of the Celestial Masters sect of Taoism, which is also known as the Way of the Five Pecks of Rice.

Southern Liang dynasty (502–557). Born in Moling, Danyang (now Nanjing, Jiangsu Province), Tao Hongjing was a well-known expert in medicine, alchemy, mathematical astronomy, geography, military strategics, sword casting, studies of Confucius Classics, literature and art and Daoism rituals. He started to read the *Shen Xian Zhuan* (Biographies of Divine Immortals) by Ge Hong[1] when he was only 10 years old. At the age of 36, he became the successor of Shangqing (Supreme Clarity) sect. Although he lived a secluded life in Mount Mao, he remained an adviser and friend to the then emperor Wu of Liang (Xiao Yan). Consequently, Tao Hongjing had the nickname Prime Minister in the Mountains.

《养性延命录》中记载："凡行气，以鼻纳气，以口吐气，微而行之名曰长息。纳气有一，吐气有六。纳气一者谓吸也，吐气六者谓吹、呼、嘻、呵、嘘、呬，皆为长息吐气之法。时寒可吹，时温可呼，委曲治病，吹以去风，呼以去热，嘻以去烦，呵以下气，嘘以散滞，呬以解极。"

The *Yang Xing Yan Ming Lu* records, 'Qi circulation can be promoted by inhaling through the nose and exhaling through the mouth. One has only one way for inhalation but six for exhalation, namely *Chui, Hu, Xi, He, Xu and hei. Chui* removes pathogenic cold or heat, *Hu* dissipates pathogenic wind and warmth, *Xi* relieves worries, *He* causes qi to descend, *Xu* resolves stagnation and *hei.* improves exhaustion .'

隋代智者大师的《童蒙止观》中用到六字诀治病，而其使用的是观想六气的方法。"但观心想，用六种气。治病者即是观能

---

1. Ge Hong (283–343), a southern official during the Jin Dynasty (263–420) of China, best known for his interest in Daoism, alchemy, and techniques of longevity.

治病。何谓六种气,一吹,二呼,三嘻,四呵,五嘘,六呬。此六种息皆于唇口之中,想心方便,转侧而作,绵微而用。颂曰:心配属呵肾属吹,脾呼肺呬圣皆知,肝藏热来嘘字至,三焦壅处但言嘻。"此处六字发音与脏腑的关系已确立。

The *Tong Meng Zhi Guan* (Samatha-vipasyana or Insight Meditation) by Master Zhiyi recorded the role of *Liu Zi Jue* in disease treatment, 'Inner visualization or insight meditation can be performed by six qi, namely *Chui, Hu, Xi, He, Xu* and *hei* ... the *He* sound is used for heart problems, the *Chui* sound for kidney problems, the *Hu* sound for spleen problems, the *hei* sound for lung problems, the *Xu* sound for liver heat and *Xi* sound for Sanjiao disorders'. Evidently, the relationship between different sounds and zang-fu organs has been established.

唐代著名道士,医药学家,被人称为"药王"的孙思邈在《备急千金药方·调气法》谓"若患心冷病,气即呼出;若热病,气即吹出。若肺病即嘘出,若肝病即呵出,若脾病即唏出,若肾病即呬出。"并主张在六字诀进行前,先做导引。

The *Bei Ji Qian Jin Yao Fang Tiao Qi Fa* (Qi Regulation Method, Important Formulas Worth a Thousand Gold Pieces for Emergency) by Sun Si-miao, a famous Daoist priest and medical expert in the Tang dynasty (618–907) (He was titled as China's King of Medicine for his significant contributions to Chinese medicine) states, 'Aspirate the *Hu* sound for heart cold and *Chui* sound for heat, aspirate the *Xu* sound for lung problems, the *He* sound for liver problems, the *Xi* sound for spleen problems and *hei* sound for kidney problems'. In addition, he believed it's essential to perform *Dao Yin* before the six healing sounds.

后世采用的导引动作,多出自唐代李奉时的《调气法》:"嘘时目瞋睁,呵时项后平叉手,呼时反托前,咽时双手擎,吹时平膝紧抱胸。"李奉时还主张按大小月编订六字诀锻炼的顺序,结合五行学说来运用六字诀。

Most *Dao Yin* movements used by later generations originated from the *Tiao Qi Fa* (Qi Regulation Method) by Li Feng-shi in the Tang dynasty, 'Keep the eyes wide open when aspirating the *Xu* sound, place the hands with crossed fingers on the occiput when aspirating the *He* sound, place the hands in front of the body when aspirating the *Hu* sound, lift the hands when aspirating the *hei* sound and squat down and lift the hands to the level of chest when aspirating the *Chui* sound'. What's more, Li Feng-shi compiled the sequence of six healing sounds according to five elements and the solar months of 30 or 31 days.

唐宣宗大中二年(848),胡愔撰的《黄庭内景五脏六腑补泻图》明确提出六字发音为"自然之理""天然之气"。书中脏腑补泻法以六字诀为主体,书中述:"肺咽、心呵、肝嘘、脾呼、肾吹、胆嘻……但为除疾,非胎息也。"《黄庭内景五脏六腑补泻图》所载的六字诀与《养性延命录》和《备急千金要方》主要在于治疗上的应用,少有养生方面的直接论述。

The *Huang Ting Nei Jing Wu Zang Liu Fu Bu Xie Tu* (Illustrations of Reinforcing and Reducing Five-Zang and Six-Fu Organs, Scripture on the Internal View of the Yellow Court) by Hu Yin during the era of emperor Xuanzong of Tang (848) clearly states that the six healing sounds are 'principles of nature' and 'qi of nature'. The text also states, 'Instead of fetal breathing (embryonic respiration), the six healing sounds are used to treat diseases: the *hei* sound for lung problems, the *He* sound for heart problems, the *Xu* sound for liver problems, the *Hu* sound for spleen problems, the *Chui* sound for kidney problems and the *Xi* sound for gallbladder problems'. According to descriptions in the *Huang*

Ting Nei Jing Wu Zang Liu Fu Bu Xie Tu, Yang Xing Yan Ming Lu and *Bei Ji Qian Jin Yao Fang*, the six healing sounds were mainly used for disease treatment. There was little information regarding their role in health cultivation.

北宋末南宋初，曾慥在其所撰《道枢》众多篇章中详细地论述了在养生保健方面的六字诀锻炼方法，并把六字诀与导引动作直接结合起来。

In the late Northern Song (960–1127) and early Southern Song (1127–1279) dynasty, Zeng Zao described the six healing sounds for health cultivation and supplemented *Dao Yin* movements in many chapters of *Dao Shu* (the Pivot of the Dao).

元代邹应博据《道藏·玉轴经》有关六字诀的记载，结合其师所授，写成《太上玉轴六字气诀》，结合定神、叩齿、漱津、存想及坐式行功，把六字诀引向静功的发展方向，兼及养生与治疗。《太上玉轴六字气诀》明代十分流行，《寿世保元》及《夷门广牍》等均有引录。

In Yuan dynasty (1271–1368), Zou Ying-bo wrote the *Tai Shang Yu Zhou Liu Zi Qi Jue* (the Great High Jade Axis Six Healing Sounds) on the basis of the literature on *Liu Zi Jue* in the *Dao Zang Yu Zhou Jing* (Scripture on Jade Axis, Daoist Canon). In his text, by integrating with mental consciousness, clicking teeth, swallowing saliva, meditation and sitting posture, *Liu Zi Jue* became a more static exercise for health cultivation and disease treatment. This text was quite popular in the Ming dynasty (1368–1644), since its contents were recorded in the *Shou Shi Bao Yuan* (Prolonging Life and Preserving the Origin) and *Yi Men Guang Du* (Extensive Records from the School of [Chen Xi] yi).

在明清时期结合导引的延年六字诀非常流行,许多气功文献都有记载,如:张三丰《张三丰太极行功歌》,胡文焕《类修要诀》,龚居中《红炉点雪》,高濂《尊生八笺》,周履靖《夷门广牍》,托名冷谦的《修龄要旨》,傅仁宇《审视瑶函》,罗洪先《万寿仙书》,徐文弼《寿世传真》等。

The *Yan Nian* (prolonging Life) *Liu Zi Jue* became very popular in the Ming and Qing (1644–1911) dynasty. They were recorded in numerous books, such as *Zhang San-feng*[1] *Tai Ji Xing Gong Ge* (Zhang San-feng Taiji Verses) by Zhang San-feng, *Lei Xiu Yao Jue* (The Essence of Categorized Exercises) by Hu Wen-huan, *Hong Lu Dian Xue* (Snow in A Red Stove, i.e., Fast Comprehension) by Gong Ju-zhong, *Zun Sheng Ba Jian* (Health Cultivation in Eight Ways) by Gao Lian, *Yi Men Guang Du* (Extensive Records from the School of [Chen Xi] yi) by Zhou lǔ-jing, *Xiu Ling Yao Zhi* (Essential Principles for Longevity) by Leng Qian, *Shen Shi Yao Han* (Collected Therapies for Eye Problems) by Fu Ren-yu, *Wan Shou Xian Shu* (Treatises on Longevity and Immortality) by Luo Hong-xian and *Shou Shi Chuan Zhen* (Treatise on Health and Longevity) by Xu Wen-bi, etc.

各家记载,都以歌诀形式(或加注)出现。歌诀有数种,最为流行的是《类修要诀》中名为《去病延年六字法》的一种,此套功法,各书辑录时,名称不一,文字也有变动,但基本精神一致。如《红炉点雪》与《审视瑶函》只录其中的"四季却病歌"及"总诀",而无"分字诀",而在每句"总诀"下祥为作注,合称《动功六字延寿诀》。《夷门广牍》所录"六气歌诀",名称与内容同《类修要诀》。在《修龄要旨》所录无总名,文字较精炼。《寿

---

1. Zhang San-feng: a legendary Chinese Taoist priest who is believed by some to have achieved immortality. He is said to have been a government official in his youth, learned Shaolin martial arts and then lived for scores of years as a Taoist priest, healer, and sage at the Wudang Mountain Taoist Temples.

世传真》有"六字行功依式样歌""六字行功应时候歌""六字行功各效验歌"等,内容与上述歌诀基本相同。

These recordings were often documented in the form of verses (or notes). The *Qu Bing* (removing diseases) *Yan Nian* (prolonging life) *Liu Zi Jue* in the *Lei Xiu Yao Jue*, among others, was the most influential one. Although it has been recorded in various names and words, its contents remained consistent. For example, the '*Si Ji Que Bing Ge* (Verses of Removing Diseases in Four Seasons)' and '*Zong Jue* (General Formula)' were recorded in the *Hong Lu Dian Xue* and *Shen Shi Yao Han*; however, '*Fen Zi Jue* (Individual Formula for Each Sound)' was not included. Instead, they made annotations for each General Formula and called them *Dong Gong Liu Zi Yan Shou Jue* (Dynamic Life-Prolonging Liu Zi Jue). The *Liu Qi Ge Jue* (Verses for Six Qi) recorded in the *Yi Men Guang Du* shared the same name and contents as that in the *Lei Xiu Yao Jue*. The verses recorded in the *Xiu Ling Yao Zhi* were simple and concise but had no collective name. The verses recorded in the *Shou Shi Chuan Zhen* shared similar contents.

以下是明清流行较广的几个口诀。

Two examples of popular *Liu Zi Jue* rhymes in Ming and Qing dynasties are as follows:

延年六字总诀

肝将嘘时目瞪睛,肺和呬气手双擎,

心呵顶上连叉手,肾吹抱取膝头平,

脾病呼时须撮口,三焦客热卧嘻宁。

General Rhyme for Yan Nian Liu Zi Jue

The liver: as you exhale with *Xu*, make sure the eyes are wide open.

The lung: as you exhale with *hei*, make sure the two hands protect the lung.

The heart: the *He* breath corresponds to the heart; cross the two hands above the head.

Chui: this matches the kidneys; wrap your arms around the knees.

For spleen symptoms: as you exhale with *Hu*, best pucker the mouth.

If heat enters Sanjiao, exhale with *Xi*.

四季却病歌

春嘘明目木扶肝，夏至呵心火自闲。

秋呬定收金肺润，肾吹惟要坎中安。

三焦嘻却除烦热，四季长呼脾化餐。

切忌出声闻口耳，其功尤胜保神丹。

Disease-Removing Rhyme in Four Seasons

In spring, breathe *Xu* to clear eyes and so wood can benefit your liver.

In summer, reach for *He* so heart-fire can be inhibited.

In fall, breathe *hei* to stabilize and gather metal, moistening the lung.

In winter, breathe *Chui* to calm kidney water.

Aspirate *Xi* to expel heat in Sanjiao.

In all four seasons take long breaths, so the spleen can process food.

And, of course, avoid exhaling noisily, not letting even your ears hear it.

This practice is even better than divine elixir.

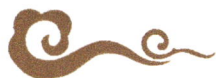

古 音 六 字 诀 • *Gu Yin Liu Zi Jue* (Six Healing Sounds)

Theoretical Foundation

理
论
基
础

古音六字诀的六个读音

Six Pronunciations of *Gu Yin Liu Zi Jue*

六字诀的发音在历史上以文字形式记录为主，明清以前，由于没有统一的汉字注音方法，读音主要靠已知之字音互切而说明。这样，就造成了人们对六字诀发音的歧义，出现了"同字不同音、同音不同字"的现象。再加上统治阶层的语系不同、文字变迁，地方口音变化等原因导致六字诀出现不同版本的发音。我们现在的普通话受北方游牧民族特别是满族的影响很大，原来的汉语方言极少卷舌的。

Historically, the pronunciations of *Liu Zi Jue* were mainly recorded in written form. Since there were no standardized phonetic annotations of Chinese characters before the Ming and Qing dynasties, the pronunciations were explained using pronunciations of other known characters. This, coupled with language families of the Ruling Class, changes of Chinese characters and regional accents, resulted in different pronunciations for the same character and same pronunciation for different characters. The mandarin today is greatly influenced by the northern nomadic people. There is little retroflex consonant in the original Chinese dialects.

六字诀正式见于陶弘景的《养性延命录》一书，而陶弘景（456—536年），属于南朝齐梁间人，其出生地在丹阳秣陵（今江苏南京），36岁时隐居茅山，是茅山派道家的代表人物，当地语音属于吴语体系。我们认为现在的苏州话与当时吴语同源，较好地保留了吴语的发音。本版本的六字诀发音则以现今苏州一带的吴语为基础。

It's known to all that *Liu Zi Jue* was first officially recorded in the *Yang Xing Yan Ming Lu* (Records on Nourishing Character & Prolonging Life) by Tao Hong-jing (456–536), a leading figure of the Maoshan School of Taoism who lived in the Southern Liang dynasty (502–557). Born in Moling, Danyang (now Nanjing, Jiangsu Province), Tao Hongjing started living in Mount Mao at the age of 36. The local pronunciation falls under the category of *Wu accent*[1], which is very similar to Suzhou accent today. Consequently, *Liu Zi Jue* pronunciations in this text are based on the *Wu* dialect.

自然发音原则是古音六字诀发音的另外一个重要原则。唐代胡愔撰的《黄庭内景五脏六腑补泻图》认为六字诀的发音是人的自然发音，明确提出六字发音为"自然之理""天然之气"，是我们生活当中不自主的发出的声音。

Natural pronunciation is another key principle for *Liu Zi Jue*. The *Huang Ting Nei Jing Zu Zang Liu Fu Bu Xie Tu* by Hu Yin in the Tang dynasty clearly states that *Liu Zi Jue* pronunciations are involuntary sounds by following the 'principle of nature' and 'qi of nature'.

现代的科学研究中，在20世纪末上海市气功研究所采用SIS95 语音识别系统来研究发音的音图特点，认为不同发音法治疗上、中、下三焦不同脏腑的疾病，这可能与发音的能量和频率有关；从上到下，能量逐渐向高频部分移动，共振峰频率也有升高的倾向。在比较了多种发音的频率后提出六字诀发音是以

---

1. *Wu* Chinese: a group of linguistically similar and historically related varieties of Chinese primarily spoken in Zhejiang province, Shanghai, and southern Jiangsu province.

江浙一带的吴音为基础,这种发音符合六字诀的发音要求,北方语发音的频率较低,能量集中于1 000 Hz以下的频段,不利于造成脏器的共振。

At the end of the 20th century, staff at the Shanghai Qigong Research Institute studied the phonetic characteristics using the SIS95 voice recognition system. They believed that different pronunciations can help to treat zang-fu disorders in upper, middle and lower *Jiao*. This might be related to their differences in energy and frequency. More specifically, from top to bottom, the energy is gradually shifted towards the high-frequency part, followed by an elevation trend of the formant frequency. They have compared frequencies of various pronunciations and concluded that *Liu Zi Jue* is more based on the *Wu* accent. The northern accent has a low frequency (the energy is more focused on the frequency band below 1,000 Hz) and is not favorable for resonance of internal organs.

下面是对每个字的发音的详解。

Explanations of each sound are as follows:

嘘

The *Xu* sound

发音为"xu"。

"xu"是人在紧张疼痛生气的情况下自然发出的声音,能疏解肝郁之气,缓解疼痛,符合《黄庭内景五脏六腑补泻图》中"肝之有疾当用嘘。嘘者肝之气……能除毁痛,皆自然之理"。

Xu is an involuntary sound when one feels pain, angry or nervous. This sound can soothe liver qi and alleviate pain.

The *Huang Ting Nei Jing Wu Zang Liu Fu Bu Xie Tu* states, 'The *Xu* sound is indicated for liver problems. It can relieve liver-qi stagnation ... and alleviate pain, which is an example of following the natural principle.'

呵
The *He* sound

发音为吴音的"喝",介于"he"与"ha"。

人在开心的状态下自然发出的声音,能让人心气条达,神清气爽。符合《黄庭内景五脏六腑补泻图》"心之有疾,当用呵,呵者,心之气⋯⋯呵能静其心,和其神。所以人之昏乱者多呵,盖天然之气也。故心病当用呵泻之也"。

He is an involuntary sound when one feels happy. It's pronounced between '*He*' and '*Ha*' in *Wu* accent. This sound can regulate heart qi and refresh the mind. The *Huang Ting Nei Jing Wu Zang Liu Fu Bu Xie Tu* states, 'The *He* sound is indicated for heart problems. It can harmonize heart qi and calm the mind. As a result, people often aspirate the *He* sound when they feel drowsy, which is an example of following the qi of nature.'

呼
The *Hu* sound

发音为"hu"。

人在胃中有热,或是吃太饱时自然会呼出胃中之气。符合《黄庭内景五脏六腑补泻图》中"脾之有疾,当用呼,呼者,脾之气⋯⋯能抽脾之疾,故人中热者,则呼以驱其弊也"。

Hu is an involuntary sound when the stomach is full or with stomach heat. The *Huang Ting Nei Jing Wu Zang Liu Fu Bu Xie Tu* states, 'The *Hu* sound is indicated for spleen problems. It can regulate spleen qi and remove stomach heat.'

哂

The *Hei* sound

发音为 "hei"。

"哂" 发音方法较多，不同的六字诀版本采用了不同的发音，主要有四种。

（1）普通话发音为 "xi"，通 "息"，与三焦 "嘻" 字诀同音。

（2）在吴音中，"息" 的发音接近 "xia" "xie"，即马礼堂养生六字诀的发音。

（3）在客家话中发音为 "si"，即健身气功六字诀的发音。

（4）在当今粤语中发音为 "hei"，即本版本的发音。

Actually this sound is pronounced as *'Hei'.*

There are mainly four pronunciations of *hei* in different versions of *Liu Zi Jue*:

Mandarin: *Xi*, same as *Xi* sound for Sanjiao.

Wu accent: *Xia* or *Xie* in *Ma Li-tang*[1] *Yang Sheng Liu Zi Jue.*

Hakka dialect: *Si*, same as the Health Qigong *Liu Zi Jue.*

Cantonese: *Hei*, used in this text.

在唐代义净三藏法师翻译的七佛药师经中有两个咒语中用到这个 "哂"，而这个咒语在藏语中的发音接近 "hei"，在宋代编订的《广韵》中 "哂" 的发音也接近 "hei"。在此我们认为

---

1. Ma Li-tang (1903–1989): a famous martial artist and dedicated to study *Liu Zi Jue* in his later years.

"hei" 的发音比较符合古代的发音方式。

The *Classics of Seven Medicine Buddha* translated by the Tripitaka Dharma Master (Yijing[1]) in the Tang dynasty used the *hei* in two incantations, which was pronounced like *Hei* in Tibetan language. The pronunciation of *hei* in *Guang Yun* (Broad Rhymes) compiled in the Song dynasty (960–1279) was also similar to *Hei.* We hereby assume the *Hei* sound is more consistent with its ancient pronunciation.

依自然发音原则，人在幽怨烦闷自然发出"咽"（hei）的声音则可以让人心情舒畅。符合《黄庭内景五脏六腑补泻图》中"肺之有疾，当用咽。咽者，肺之气也……能抽肺之疾，所以人之有怨气填塞胸臆者，则长咽而泻之，盖自然之理也。"在此我们认为"hei"的发音比较符合古代的发音方式。

By following the natural Vocalization principle, *Hei* is an involuntary sound when one feels unhappy or worried. This sound can make you feel good. The *Huang Ting Nei Jing Wu Zang Liu Fu Bu Xie Tu* states, 'The *Hei* sound is indicated for lung problems. It can regulate lung qi ... and remove lung problems. It's natural that people aspirate the syllabus of *Hei* when they have hard feelings. This is an example of following the principle of nature'.

吹
The *Chui* sound

发音为吴音的"吹"，不卷舌。

---

1. Yijing (635–713): a Tang period monk originally from Shandong. He traveled to India to study Buddhism, leaving in 671 and returning in 695. During his 25 year stay, he gathered many Sanskrit texts. Later, he translated some 50 texts.

人在寒冷、气机沉滞不通时会自然牙关紧张，在此口型下的发音即是吴音的"吹"，发音接近"ci"。符合《黄庭内景五脏六腑补泻图》中"肾之有疾，当用吹，吹者，肾之气⋯⋯能抽肾之疾，故人有积气冲臆者，则强吹也，肾气沉滞不通时，重吹则渐通也"。

Chui is pronounced in Wu accent and does not involve tongue rolling. It is an involuntary sound of tight jaw when one feels cold or qi stagnation. The pronunciation is similar to ci. The *Huang Ting Nei Jing Wu Zang Liu Fu Bu Xie Tu* states, 'The *Chui* sound is indicated for kidney problems. It can harmonize kidney qi ... and remove kidney problems. Therefore forceful *Chui* sounds can help to disperse qi, and deep *Chui* sounds can unblock kidney qi'.

嘻

The *Xi* sound

发音为"xi"。

人在全身舒畅时发出"嘻"的声音。也就是笑嘻嘻的时候发出的"嘻"字音。《黄庭内景五脏六腑补泻图》曰："鼻渐长引气，以口嘻之，去胆家病，并除阴脏一切冷。"

Xi is an involuntary sound when one feels happy, comfortable and smiles. The *Huang Ting Nei Jing Wu Zang Liu Fu Bu Xie Tu* states 'Inhaling with the nose and exhaling with the *Xi* sound from the mouth can alleviate gollbladder problems and remove cold retention in zang organs'.

流传较广的六字诀读音版本

Common Pronunciation Versions of *Liu Zi Jue*

目前社会上流传较广的有"养气功六字诀""峨眉派六字诀""六字真言""健身气功六字诀"。

At present, there are four popular pronunciation versions of *Liu Zi Jue*, namely, *Ma Li-tang Yang Qi Gong Liu Zi Jue, E Mei Pai*[1] *Liu Zi Jue, Liu Zi Zhen Yan* and *Jian Shen Qi Gong Liu Zi Jue*.

马礼堂的"养生六字诀"的六个发音分别为：嘘：读"xū"；呵：读"kē"；呼：读"hū"；呬：读"xia"或"xie"；吹：读"chuī"；嘻：读"xī"。

Pronunciations of *Ma Li-tang Yang Sheng Liu Zi Jue*: xū, kē, hū, xia or xie, chui and xī.

健身气功六字诀的发音为：嘘：读"xū"；呵：读"hē"；呼：读"hū"；呬：读"si"；吹：读"chuī"；嘻：读"xī"。

Pronunciations of *Health Qigong Liu Zi Jue*: xū, hē, hū, si, chui and xī.

不同版本的六字诀在发音上虽然存在出入，但在实践应用中都表现出了良好医疗养生保健作用。

Despite the slight differences in pronunciation, various versions of *Liu Zi Jue* share similar effect in medical treatment

---

1. The E Mei Sect is a fictional martial arts sect named after the place where it is based, Mount E Mei.

and health cultivation.

六字诀发声与不发声的不同功用
Functions of Voicing or Voiceless *Liu Zi Jue*

六字诀是吐纳法的一种，关于发出声音和不发出声音在历史上也有不同的论述。

Liu Zi Jue is a subtype of breathing exercise. Historically, there are different discourses regarding whether they are voicing or voiceless.

陶弘景《养性延命录》曾述："常以鼻引气，口中吐气，当令气声逐字吹、呼、嘘、呵、唏、呬吐之。"从"气声逐字"来看陶弘景的发声为"气声"。以发音方式来讲，气声是一种让气流通过未完全振动的声带时发出的声音，不是我们平时用声带振动发出的喉音。

The *Yang Xing Yan Ming Lu* by Tao Hong-jing states, 'Inhale through the nose, exhale through the mouth and aspirate the sounds of *Chui, Hu, Xu, He, Xi* and *hei* one by one with qi'. Unlike guttural sounds through vocal cord vibration, here it means breathing sound — a sound produced by air flowing through incompletely vibrated vocal cord.

隋代天台高僧智者大师的《修习止观坐禅法要》提到了六字诀的发声方式："此六种息皆于唇口中，想心方便，转侧而坐，绵微而用。"主张使用观想的方法。

The *Xiu Xi Zhi Guan Zuo Chan Fa Yao* (Essential Principles

for Sitting Meditation) by Zhiyi, an eminent Tiantai[1] monk mentioned that, 'the six breathing sounds are made through the lips and mouth ...' and proposed using contemplation method.

唐代孙思邈在其《养生歌》中提到"切忌出声闻口耳,其功犹胜保身丹"。之后,基本都主张发声勿令耳闻,恐气泄耳。胡愔撰《黄庭内景五脏六腑补泻图》中"以鼻微长引气,以口咽之,勿令耳闻。""以鼻微长引气,以口呵之,皆调气如上,勿令自耳闻之"。主张吐气勿令耳闻。

The *Yang Sheng Ge* (Rhymes for Health Cultivation) by Sun Si-miao in the Tang dynasty mentioned that, 'six breathing inaudible sounds are better than life-preserving elixirs'. Ever since then, it has been generally accepted to aspirate inaudible sounds. The *Huang Ting Nei Jing Wu Zang Liu Fu Bu Xie Tu* by Hu Yin states, 'to inhale through the nose and aspirate inaudible *hei* sound with the mouth'.

元代邹应博的《太上玉轴六字气诀》要求吐气和吸气都不发声,认为发声则损气。如:"先念呵字,以吐心中毒气,念时耳不得闻呵字声,闻即气粗,乃损心气也;念毕,仰头闭口,以鼻徐徐吸天地之清气,以补心气,吸时耳亦不得闻吸声,闻即气粗,亦损心气也。"

The *Tai Shang Yu Zhou Liu Zi Qi Jue* by Zou Yin-bo in the Yuan dynasty proposes no sound in exhalation or inhalation, assuming that sound impairs qi, 'Aspirate the *He* sound first to remove toxic qi in the heart; however, do not make audible *He* sound, since this (audible sound results from fast breathing) may damage heart qi. After this, raise the head with the mouth

---

1. An important school of Buddhism in China, Japan, Korea, and Vietnam, revering the Lotus Sutra as the highest teaching in Buddhism.

closed and inhale fresh air to supplement heart qi; however, do not make audible inhaling sound, since this may also damage heart qi'.

清代康熙年间的《寿世青编》中载有"静功六字却病法"，记载吐气发音须轻声："假如春月，须低声念嘘字，不可令耳闻，闻即气粗，粗恐气泄耳。"

The *Shou Shi Qing Bian* (Collections of Qigong Practice for Health Cultivation) in Kangxi era (1661–1722) of the Qing dynasty recorded the *Jing Gong Liu Zi Que Bing Fa* (static six word disease-removing method) and states, 'pronounce the *Xu* sound in a low voice and do not make the sound audible, since audible sound results from fast breathing and fast breathing may con sume qi.'

马礼堂的"养生六字诀"主张先期需要发声排除浊气，学会后呼吸、发音变得轻些，后来仅有气流出入，发音而变为无声。

Ma Li-tang believed it's necessary to aspirate the sound to remove turbid qi at first, then gradually use voiceless breathing'.

20世纪末上海市气功研究所对六字诀发音的音图研究中认为，六字诀的正确发音应该是声带不振动的方式，其能量来自空气经过口腔的腔体振动，而不是声带振动。声带振动的发音能量集中于1 000 Hz以下的频段，不利于造成脏器的共振。要求在吸气和吐气中以轻声为主，包含唇音、齿音和各腔体共振音，不发喉音，发音中通过口型、气压、共振等调节相应的脏腑部位。

At the end of the 20th century, staff at the Shanghai Qigong

Research Institute studied the phonation of *Liu Zi Jue* and concluded that the vocal cord vibration should not be involved in correct phonation. Instead of vocal cord vibration, the energy of *Liu Zi Jue* comes from the cavity vibration. The phonation energy of vocal cord vibration is focused on the frequency band below 1,000 Hz and not favorable for resonance of internal organs. Therefore, soft voice including labial sound, dental sound and cavity resonance sound (no guttural sound) are involved in inhalation and exhalation. Furthermore, different zang-fu organs are regulated by the shape of the mouth, air pressure and resonance.

21世纪初的"健身气功六字诀"采用的是出声发音的方法。

In the beginning of the 21st century, voicing was adopted by health qigong *Liu Zi Jue*.

总而言之，陶弘景的六字诀是为了泻气实治病，故采用了气声的方法。后世的六字诀多用于养生恐气泄，故采用勿令耳闻的方法。在具体实践应用中可根据具体情况而又所别。

In summary, the *Liu Zi Jue* by Tao Hong-jing adopted qi sound to reduce pathogenic factors. *Liu Zi Jue* by the later generations used inaudible sounds to preserve qi and promote health.

古音六字诀与五行

Gu Yin Liu Zi Jue and Five Elements

天给人吸食五气，地给人食五味。五气入鼻，藏于心肺，它使人的五色修明,声音响亮;五味入口,藏于肠胃,能养五气,气各而生,津液相生,精神也就充沛。人作为受天地养育的生命,本身就是大自然的一个组成部分,与天地的运行状态息息相关。人因自身的贪求失去了与天地之间的和谐感应,而在气功锻炼中的"天人合一",则是让人回归自然之道。

The heaven provides us with five qi, and the earth provides us with five flavors. The five qi enter through the nose and are stored in the heart and lung, enabling five colors to be bright and our voices to be loud and clear. The five flavors enter through the mouth and are stored in the intestines and stomach, nourishing the five qi and body fluids and making us energetic. As an inseparable part of the nature, human life is closely associated with the heaven and earth. Sometimes one loses the harmonious interaction with the heaven and earth. The 'unity of man and nature' in qigong practice can help man return to the nature.

六字诀发音中的前五音与五脏相对应,而五脏又和五行相对应,《素问·阴阳应象大论》中详细阐述了五行的对应关系,这使得古音六字诀在锻炼过程中可以配合诸多的元素,以增强锻炼效果。如练功中配合五音,每一节对应不同的方位,不同季节练习不同字诀等,是古代常有的方法。

Of the six healing sounds, the first five are corresponding to five zang organs. The *Su Wen Yin Yang Ying Xiang Da Lun* (chapter 5 of the Basic Questions) explained the correlation between five zang organs and five elements. As a result, multiple elements can be combined in practicing *Gu Yin Liu Zi Jue* to enhance the beneficial effect. It's very common in ancient past to combine five notes, directions and seasons into different sounds.

五行对照
Combination of Five Elements, Notes, Directions and Seasons

发音	嘘	呵	呼	呬	吹
五脏	肝	心	脾	肺	肾
五行	木	火	土	金	水
五音	角	徵	宫	商	羽
五方	东	南	中	西	北
季节	春	夏	长夏	秋	冬

Five sounds	Xu	He	Hu	hei	Chui
Five zang organs	Liver	Heart	Spleen	Lung	Kidney
Five elements	Wood	Fire	Earth	Metal	Water
Five notes	Jiao	Zheng	Gong	Shang	Yu
Five directions	East	South	Central	West	North
Five seasons	Spring	Summer	Late summer	Autumn	Winter

在古音六字诀的锻炼中，我们采用的五行相生的顺序，而在历史上也有使用五行相克的方法，多用于疾病治疗。

During practice of *Gu Yin Liu Zi Jue*, five elements are often combined by the sequence of mutual promotion. Historically, they were also combined by the sequence of mutual inhibition for disease treatment.

五行相生：相生就是相互促进，相互资生的意思，表述的是事物之间的相互联系和相互影响。其具体关系为木生火，火生土，土生金，金生水，水生木。

Mutually promoted relationships are as follows: wood promotes fire, fire promotes earth, earth promotes metal, metal promotes water and water promotes wood.

五行相克：相克就是相互抑制，相互制约的意思，表述的是事物间的相互作用的表现。其具体关系为木克土，土克水，水克火，火克金，金克木。

Mutually inhibited relationships are as follows: wood inhibits earth, earth inhibits water, water inhibits fire, fire inhibits metal and metal inhibits wood.

古音六字诀与五音
Gu Yin Liu Zi Jue and Five Notes

在我们中医学理论中，五脏可以影响五音，五音可以调节五脏。《黄帝内经》中把"宫商角徵羽"五音与五脏相配，用五音可以调节五脏：脾应宫，其声漫而缓；肺应商，其声促以清；肝应角，其声呼以长；心应徵，其声雄以明；肾应羽，其声沉以细，此为五脏正音。

In Chinese medicine, five zang organs can affect five notes and five notes can regulate five zang organs. The *Huang Di Nei Jing* (Yellow Emperor's Internal Classic) matches five notes with five zang organs: *Gong* (slow) with the spleen, *Shang* (abrupt) with the lung, *Zheng* (strong) with the heart, *Jiao* (long) with the liver and *Yu* (deep, thready) with the kidney'.

五音也有归经、升降浮沉、寒热温凉，可以感染、调理情绪，进而影响身体。在聆听中让曲调与情志、脏腑之气产生共鸣，达到疏通经脉、通畅精神和防病养生的作用。若加以运用五行原理，五音的相生、相克、相互制约关系，可以演化出诸多的辩证应用方式。

Five notes have the property of ascending, descending, (cool) cold and (warm) heat and enter different meridians. They can influence or regulate emotions. Harmony among notes, emotions and qi of zang-fu organs can unblock meridians, benefit emotion and promote health. Specific applications can evolve from the mutual promotion and inhibition interactions among five elements and notes.

五音让现代人有些陌生,然博古家们用现代音乐予以解释。

Five notes may seem strange in modern society. However, they can be explained in the perspective of modern music.

角音:具有"木"之特性,可入肝,相当于简谱中的"3"。角调式乐曲:有大地回春,万物萌生,生机盎然的旋律,曲调亲切爽朗。

Jiao note has the property of wood and enters the liver. It can be understood as '3' in numbered musical notation. *Jiao*-note music is often cheerful, representing the ideas of rebirth, rejuvenation and regrowth of everything in the season of spring.

徵音:具有"火"之特性,可入心,相当于简谱中的"5"。徵调式乐曲:热烈欢快,活泼轻松,构成层次分明,性情欢畅的气氛。

Zheng note has the property of fire and enters the heart. It can be understood as '5' in numbered musical notation. *Zheng*-note music is often lively and merry.

宫音:具有"土"之特性,可入脾,相当于简谱中的"1"。宫调式乐曲:风格悠扬沉静,淳厚庄重。

Gong note has the property of earth and enters the spleen. It can be understood as '1' in numbered musical notation. *Gong*-note music is often melodious, profound and solemn.

商音：具有"金"之特性，可入肺，相当于简谱中的"2"。商调式乐曲：风格高亢悲壮，铿锵雄伟。

Shang note has the property of metal and enters the lung. It can be understood as '2' in numbered musical notation. *Shang*-note music is often loud, moving and sonorous.

羽音：具有"水"之特性，可入肾，相当于简谱中的"6"。羽调式乐曲：风格清纯，凄切哀怨，苍凉柔润，如天垂晶幕，行云流水。

Yu note has the property of water and enters the kidney. It can be understood as '6' in numbered musical notation. *Yu*-note music is often pure, sad, desolate and soft, like floating clouds and flowing water.

古音六字诀的六个发音中的前五个对应相应的五音，嘘为角音，呵为徵音，呼为宫音，呬为商音，吹为羽音。从五脏和身体部位来讲，胸腹的音调较低，两胁略高，背部和腰部较高，这个频率不同与振动所需的压力有关。嘻不纳入五音范围，在20世纪末上海市气功研究所对六字诀发音的振动频率做过的研究中发现，嘻的频率比前五音还要高，相当于简谱中的"7"。

Of the six healing sounds (*Liu Zi Jue*), the first five sounds correspond with the five notes — *Xu* with *Jiao*, *He* with *Zheng*, *Hu* with *Gong, hei* with *Shang and Chui* with *Yu*. In terms of the five-zang organs and body parts, tones from the chest and abdomen are lower, tones from the rib areas are slightly higher and tones from the back and waist are even higher. This frequency is associated with the pressure for vibration.

The *Xi* sound is not covered in five notes. Studies on vibration frequency of *Xi* found that it had a higher frequency than the first five sounds and can be understood as '7' in numbered musical notation.

古音六字诀与十二经脉
Gu Yin Liu Zi Jue and Twelve Regular Meridians

十二经脉是经络系统的主体,具有表里经脉相合,与相应脏腑络属的主要特征。十二经脉的循行走向:手三阴经从胸走手,手三阳经从手走头,足三阳经从头走足,足三阴经从足走腹(胸)。在古音六字诀的导引动作中需要牵拉和锻炼相应的经络,掌握经络的走向有助于准确地把握导引动作。

The twelve regular meridians are the major part of the meridian system. They connect internally with the zang-fu organs and externally with the surface of the body. As for the pathways of the twelve regular meridians, three hand-yin meridians travel from the chest to the hand, three hand-yang meridians travel from the hand to the head, three foot-yang meridians travel from the head to the foot and three foot-yin meridians travel from the foot to the abdomen (chest). It's essential to be familiar with the pathways of meridians since different meridians need to be pulled and exercised in *Dao Yin* movements of *Gu Yin Liu Zi Jue.*

古音六字诀的导引动作与经络关系密切。"呬"字诀动作以手太阴肺经和手阳明大肠经为导引。"呼"字诀动作以足阳明胃经和足太阴脾经为导引。"呵"字诀动作以手少阴心经和手太阳小肠经为导引。"吹"字诀动作以足少阴肾经和足太阳膀胱经为导引。"嘻"字诀动作以手少阳三焦经和手厥阴心包经为导引。"嘘"字诀动作以足少阳胆经和足厥阴肝经为导引。

For example, the *Dao Yin* movements of *hei* sound are guided by lung meridian of hand-Taiyin and large intestine meridian of hand-Yangming, the *Dao Yin* movements of *Hu* sound by stomach meridian of foot-Yangming and spleen meridian of foot-Taiyin, the *Dao Yin* movements of *He* sound by heart meridian of hand-Shaoyin and small intestine meridian of hand-Taiyang, the *Dao Yin* movements of *Chui* sound by kidney meridian of foot-Shaoyin and bladder meridian of foot-Taiyang, the *Dao Yin* movements of *Xi* sound by Sanjiao meridian of hand-Shaoyang and pericardium meridian of hand-Jueyin, and *Dao Yin* movements of *Xu* sound by gallbladder meridian of foot-Shaoyang and liver meridian of foot-Jueyin.

十二经脉循行图见"经络图"。

Please see annex for distribution and pathways of twelve regular meridians.

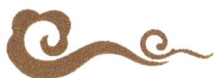

Characteristics and Essential Principles

特色与要领

功 法 特 色
Characteristics of *Liu Zi Jue*

吐故纳新
Exhaling the Old and Inhaling the New

通过声音和气息调整身体状态是六字诀的最大特色，在陶弘景记载的六字诀中甚至只用了吐纳之法，而无导引动作。其通过特定的口型、不同的发声方法来调整身体相应部位气机的开合升降，进而达到调整脏腑气机平衡的作用。本六字诀沿用了吴音的发音口型和自然发声的原则，使得发音自然。

Liu Zi Jue is mainly characterized by harmonizing the body through voice and breathing. The *Liu Zi Jue* recorded by Tao Hong-jing only mentioned *Tu* (breathing out) *Na* (breathing in) method (no *Dao Yin* movements). By specific shapes of the lips and vocalization, *Liu Zi Jue* can regulate opening, closing, ascending and descending of corresponding body parts and thus harmonize qi activities of the zang-fu organs. *Liu Zi Jue* in this text adopted the lip shapes of the *Wu* accent and natural vocalization.

循经导引
Meridian Guiding & Stretching

本六字诀沿用了明代流行的延年六字诀的动作口诀，每节动作都有相应的经络作为导引，意境分明，习练者只要了解相应经络的大致走向，在操作中拔伸牵拉相应部位，很容易把握其操作要领。

Liu Zi Jue in this text used the *Dao Yin* movements in *Yan Nian Liu Zi Jue* of the Ming dynasty. Each movement is guided and stretched by different meridians. It's easy to stretch and pull relevant body parts as long as one knows the general pathways of meridians.

意气相随
Coordination between Mind and Qi

六字诀的锻炼讲究内气的调整，对意念清静度的要求较高。需要以意领气、意气相随，表现为身体整体性的开合升降，动作缓慢柔和，圆转如意，婉转连绵。在操作中配合情绪意境调节，使得六字诀的锻炼对情绪的调整有独特的作用。

Since *Liu Zi Jue* focuses on regulating internal qi, a tranquil mind is highly demanded. It's important to use mind to guide qi, manifesting as, closing, ascending and descending of the body as a whole and slow, gentle, uninterrupted movements like floating clouds and flowing water. In this way, *Liu Zi Jue* can regulate our emotions.

适用面广
Wide Application

本功法根据习练的不同层次可以逐层深入，逐步变换发声方式和呼吸方式，在身体操作上可以逐步加入提肛、开背、开胯等元素，其外形动作简单易学，然其内涵操作无有止境，使得六字诀的锻炼不仅适合入门功法操作，也适合深层次的锻炼。

Although *Liu Zi Jue* seems easy to learn for beginners, it has profound implications. Over time, those who practice can go deeper by changing the way they vocalize and breathe and adding extra movements such as lifting up the anus, opening up the back and hip joints.

功 法 要 领
Essential Principles of *Liu Zi Jue*

松紧结合
Combined Relaxation and Tightening

松不仅是身体的，更重要的是心意上的。没有心意上的松没法做到身体上的彻底放松，在身体上松也有不同的境界，一直要松到韧带、关节，甚至是身体深层次的部位。紧则是在松的基础上，动作中如提肛敛臀、握固等都是紧的操作。如此一松一紧，有阴有阳，则气机通畅。

It's important to relax the mind as well as body, because one cannot thoroughly relax the body without relaxing the mind. Relaxation of the body involves the ligaments, joints and deeper parts. It's also important to tighten during lifting up the anus, tucking the buttocks in and firm gripping. Combined relaxation and tightening can balance yin and yang and circulate qi.

轻柔和缓
Softness and Moderation

锻炼中以内气引导带动外形的变化，动作轻柔，不僵不拘，轻松自如，舒展大方，节奏和缓，动作如行云流水般的流畅，身体没有僵硬之处，与体育锻炼的肌肉型动作相区别。

Unlike muscular movements in physical exercise, *Liu Zi Jue* uses internal qi to guide the body, manifesting as soft, gentle and relaxed movements.

圆活整体
Three-dimensional Rounded Movements

动作路线圆活带有弧形，不起楞角，不顶不丢，不僵不滞，灵活自如，顺势应变。身体以下丹田为中心，整体性开合升降，一气呵成，节节贯穿，无断续之处。

Instead of rough edges and stiffness or rigidity, *Dao Yin* movements of *Liu Zi Jue* are rounded, flexible, adaptable (change with ease) and uninterrupted. Using the lower Dantian as the pivot, the body opens, closes, ascends and descends as a whole.

内外兼修
Internal and External Cultivation

内修关系到气的质，是宽大的还是狭隘的，是明畅的还是阴暗的，是柔和的还是刚猛的，是宁静的还是躁动的，是和气的还是冲撞的等，这些都是要靠内修来调整。如果练了一身浊气只会伤人伤己。内修好的人，气机柔和通畅，意念清净，可以意到气到，其所练之气也不是后天浊气，而是先天真气。《黄帝内经》中讲"恬淡虚无，真气从之"，孟子也有"吾善养浩然正气"的说法。

Internal cultivation decides the quality of qi—broad-minded or narrow-minded, bright or dull, soft or hard, tranquil or agitated, gentle or aggressive. Turbid qi hurts oneself as well as others. Through internal cultivation, one can have smooth qi circulation and a peaceful mind and thus accumulate genuine qi. Just like the quotation from the *Huang Di Nei Jing*, 'genuine qi will be with you when you achieve Tian (peaceful joy), Dan (no greed for fame and wealth), Xu (void) and Wu (nothingness)'. Mencius also mentioned, 'I'm good at nourishing my flood-like righteous qi ...'

炼养相兼
Combined Exercise and Nourishment

通过养气才有可练的气，否则练气犹如空锅烧水，会把锅都烧坏的。在古音六字诀锻炼中情志调养、饮食调养、起居调养是古音六字诀气机运行的基础。因情志对气机影响甚大，在古音六字诀的锻炼中必不可缺。《素问·举痛论》"怒则气上、喜则气缓、悲则气消、恐则气下、惊则气乱、思则气结"讲的就是七情对气血的影响，同样人的欲望使得我们的气化火而消耗。古音六字诀的锻炼以呼吸吐纳带动气机运行，需要习练者心平气和，避免情志的大起大落，特别是怒、欲、思的调节，否则容易出现气机的混乱甚至走火入魔。

If we burn an empty pot (without water) on fire, the pot will definitely be burnt out. Likewise, we need to nourish qi for exercise. Regulation of emotion, diet and daily living serves as the foundation of smooth qi circulation. Since emotions can greatly affect qi activity, it's essential to regulate emotions during exercise of *Gu Yin Liu Zi Jue*. The *Su Wen Ju Tong Lun* (Chapter 39 of the Basic Questions) states, 'Anger causes qi to ascend, joy causes qi to slow down, sorrow causes qi to disperse, fear causes qi to disorder and worry causes qi to stagnate'. Greed causes qi to transform into fire, which in turn consumes qi of the body. Qi activity during exercise of *Gu Yin Liu Zi Jue* is guided by breathing, it is important to keep a peaceful mind and avoid anger, greed and worry. Otherwise qi disorder or even qigong deviation (*Zou Huo Ru Mo* literally means catching fire entering demon and actually means go insane) may develop.

循序渐进
Step by Step

六字诀的操作有浅有深，在习练过程中要稳步深入，循序渐进，不可好高骛远。没有前面的基础，勉强做高要求的操作只会导致身心的不协调，因为练功是个不断积累的过程，功效是随着练功时间的进程而逐步显现出来的。在功效上，随着功夫的深入会越显效果，我们在锻炼中要有"只顾攀登莫问山高"的精神。功效的获得，都是由小到大，由微至著。由于练功者体质、病情和掌握练功方法的程度不同，故其获效的时间长短不一。气功的实践性很强，要靠遵循锻炼的原则，经过长期苦练，才能求得正果。

For *Liu Zi Jue* exercise, it's necessary to go step by step. Reaching for what is beyond your grasp without a good foundation may result in body-mind incoordination. The beneficial effect of *Liu Zi Jue* exercise increases with time. However, the time-effect relationship varies due to one's constitution, health condition and exercise skill. Just like other forms of qigong, *Liu Zi Jue* is very practical and the spirit of 'climbing a tall mountain without asking its height' is highly needed.

注重呼吸、时辰、练功禁忌
Respiration, Timing and Contraindications

在呼吸上,对于初练者要自然呼吸,不可强求腹式、逆腹式呼吸等,以免引起不适。在发声上不可追求声大,免得耗气泄气过多。随着不断的操作,锻炼者的呼吸形式,气机调节能力等都会逐步地改善。

It's advisable for beginners to use natural breathing. Abdominal or reverse abdominal breathing may cause discomfort. In addition, do not pursue loud sounds during exercise, since they may consume qi. The breathing, mental regulation and qi activity will improve with time.

作为养生效果,古音六字诀发声中要求吐气缓慢,可在嘴前放置纸张或棉球等轻物,以不被明显吹动为好。大吹大呼者只适用于泻实邪。《元道经》曰:"鼻引口吐,不可排积元气,而可以去浮寒客热而已。"特别对于虚者,练习时要注意发音勿令耳闻,同时也可以配合药食补法。胡文焕的《养生导引法》说:"主治六经本病之邪也。然五脏不足,又在药食气味为补。"

For the purpose of health cultivation, a slow exhalation is required for *Gu Yin Liu Zi Jue*: place a piece of paper or cotton ball in front of the mouth and exhalation does not cause noticeable moving of the paper or cotton ball. Big fast exhalation is only used to reduce excessive pathogenic factors. The *Yuan Dao Jing* (A novel about how ordinary people become immortals) states, 'Inhale with the nose and exhale with the mouth, but do not exhale the yuan-primordial qi and just get rid of superficial cold or heat'. For people with a weak constitution (deficiency), it's particularly important not to make audible sounds. The *Yang Sheng Dao Yin Fa* (Health Cultivation & Dao Yin Methods) by Hu Wen-huan records, 'six healing sounds are mainly used to reduce pathogenic factors in six meridians; whereas medicated food can be used for deficiency of the five-zang organs'.

对于古音六字诀锻炼的时辰，一般主张在子时之后午时之前，也就是中午之前，如《备急千金要方·养性》中记载："凡调气之法，夜半后日中前，气生得调。日中后夜半前，气死不得调。"此段时间属阳气生发之时，认为吸入的气质较好。在历史上也有按不同时辰、不同月份季节、不同方位加以配合练习，比较复杂，不适合日常操作。在《养性延命录》有"天恶风猛、大寒大热时，勿取气"之文，是告诫不要在天气剧烈变化与气温过高、过低的情况下进行六字诀锻炼。

It's generally believed that exercise of *Gu Yin Liu Zi Jue* is better performed before noon. The *Bei Ji Qian Jin Yao Fang Yang Xing* (Cultivation of Character, Important Formulas Worth a Thousand Gold Pieces for Emergency) states, 'qi can be regulated from midnight to noon but not the other way around'. Historically, *Shi Chen*[1] (time), months and directions were also taken into consideration for *Liu Zi Jue* exercise. However, they are too complicated and not operational. The *Yang Xing Yan*

---

1. one of the 12 two-hour periods into which the day was traditionally divided

Ming Lu states, 'Do not try moving qi in cold windy or extremely hot days'.

　　练功前后要遵守的常规注意事项有情绪安宁、身体调整舒适、衣着宽松、避风口等。要强调的是古音六字诀在锻炼前后三天避免房事，因其为内气运行之法，在房事空虚后运行内气，犹如空锅烧水，对锻炼身体无益甚至反而有害。用于疾病治疗者需特别注意。

　　Finally, before and after exercise, it's advisable to maintain a peaceful mind, stay comfortable, wear loose clothes and avoid wind. It's worth noting that sex needs to be avoided two days before and after exercise of *Gu Yin Liu Zi Jue*, because like burning a pot without water, moving internal qi after sex can be harmful to the body. This is especially important for disease treatment.

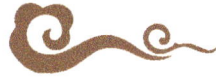

古 音 六 字 诀　·　*Gu Yin Liu Zi Jue* (Six Healing Sounds)

Movements of *Liu Zi Jue*

功法操作

基 础 操 作
Basic Movements

发声操作
Vocalization

在教学实践应用中，采取不同的发声方式有不同的效果，不同的练功层次采用不同的发声方式，不同体质的人采用不同的发声方式。本古音六字诀的发声方式以下几种。

Teaching practice has proven that different vocalization methods can produce different effects. People with different levels or constitutions can have different vocalization methods. This text contains the following four methods:

1. 默念法
1. Silent speech

有口型，动口唇，但不出声或轻出声。
其特点为不泄气，适合气虚者、初练者等。
Method: Moving of lips/mouth but no or soft sounds.
Characteristics: Preserving qi.
Applicable objects: Beginners or those with qi deficiency.

2. 默想法
2. Meditated speech

需要一定的观想基础，不动口型，不发声，感觉相应的字音在脑海、体内及周围环绕，犹如听完音乐会后仍能听到音乐在脑中余音缭绕的感觉。

Method: No moving of the lips/mouth but perception of the sounds in the mind, inside the body and surrounding environment, like lingering musical sound after a concert.

其特点为通过对相应音声的观想引导内在气机的整体性调整。适合有一定的观想基础者。

Characteristics: Use visualization to guide internal qi activity.

Applicable objects: Those who practiced meditation.

3. 气声法
3. Qi speech

以吐气为主，不发喉音，有明显的吹气感和吹气声，可表现为唇音、齿音、喉音、牙音、舌音。

Method: Mainly exhalation (no vocalization of guttural sound) and obvious blowing sensation and sound, manifesting as labial sound, dental sound, guttural sound, tooth sound and tongue sound.

气声法以吹吐气为主，用于实证泻法，体虚者不可使用。

Characteristics: Blowing and exhaling qi

Applicable objects: Those with a strong body constitution or excessive syndrome.

4. 腔体共振法
4. Cavity resonance

腔体共振法需要在身体放松的基础上才能做到，发声音的时候不发喉音，以身体的一定部位作为共振腔，带动身体产生共振的低频音，其特色为声音轻柔低沉浑厚，有磁性感，可以起到轻柔振动全身气脉的作用，犹如文火炖汤。腔体共振法不适合初练者习练，必须在老师的指导下练习。切忌不可盲求振动力度反而振伤脏腑经脉。

Method: With a fully relaxed body (no vocalized guttural sound), use certain body parts as the resonance cavity to guide the body to produce a low frequency sound.

Characteristics: Sounds are soft, deep, vigorous and magnetic. These sounds can gently vibrate meridians, like simmering soup over a slow fire.

This method needs instructions of the teacher and not recommended for beginners. Caution: Over-vibration may impair zang-fu organs and meridians.

总而言之，初学者适用默念法，其他的发声形式需在老师的指导下进行相应操作，以免掌握不当产生不好的作用。在六字诀的发声过程中若主动吐气，有明显吹气感为泻法，虚证者不可多吐气。虚证者和初练者以默念、默想法为主，吐气宜缓慢柔和。习练有素者可采用腔体共振法的方式。

In summary, beginners are advised to use silent speech method.

Instructions of the teacher are necessary for other methods. During vocalization exercise, active exhalation with an obvious blowing sensation is used for excessive syndrome only. Beginners and those with a deficient syndrome are advised to use silent speech or meditated speech, coupled with slow soft exhalation. Those with accumulated experience can try the cavity resonance method.

口型操作
Lips/mouth Shape

六字诀的发声有以上多种，但口型是一定的，不同的口型会产生不同的压力，从而对不同的脏器部位产生作用，特别在发腔体共振音时相应部位会有较明显的振动感。

Different shapes of the lips/mouth can produce different pressures and work on different body parts and zang-fu organs. Cavity resonance vocalization can also produce vibration in certain body parts.

1. 嘘字口型
1. The lips/mouth shape of *Xu* sound

嘘字口型是人在紧张疼痛生气的情况下自然发出的声音，该口型自然带动两胁部位。发音为"xu"。

Xu is an involuntary sound when one feels pain, nervous or angry. The rib areas are involved in aspirating this sound.

双唇微微闭合，上下齿之留有缝隙，嘴角向两侧引，有张开

Shape of the lips/mouth: Slightly pucker the lips, allow some space between the upper and lower teeth, pull the mouth corners to both sides (to open up the rib areas) and extend the tip of the tongue forward. The aspiration comes out through the space between the teeth and both sides of the tongue.

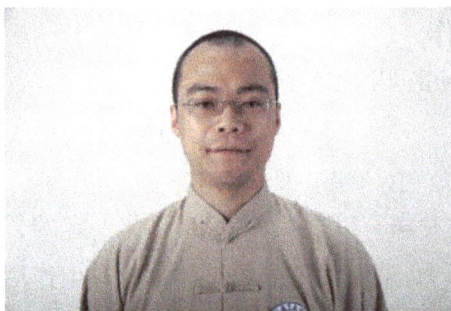

嘘字口型图　　The lips/mouth shape of *Xu* sound

2. 呵字口型
2. The lips/mouth shape of *He* sound

呵字口型是人在开心的状态下自然发出的笑声。该口型自然带动胸背部。发吴音"喝"，介于"he"与"ha"。

He is an involuntary sound when one feels happy. The chest and back are involved in aspirating this sound. In *Wu* accent, the *He* sound is between *He* and *Ha*.

唇齿半张，两腮稍有后拉，有打开后背之意，舌体微微后缩并上拱，舌贴于下颚，气从舌上与上腭之间缓缓而出。

Shape of the lips/mouth: Make the lips and teeth half open,

slightly pull the cheeks backward (to open up the back), retract the tongue body and curl up to touch the lower palate. The aspiration slowly comes out through the space between the tongue and upper palate.

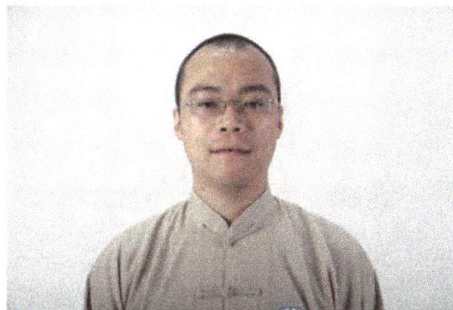

呵字口型图　　The lips/mouth shape of *He* sound

3. 呼字口型
3. The lips/mouth shape of *Hu* sound

　　呼字口型是人在胃中有热，或是吃太饱时自然会呼出胃中之气。该口型可松开食道，自然带动胃脘部位。发音为"hu"。

Hu is an involuntary sound when one has stomach heat or feels full after eating food. Aspirating this sound can relax the esophagus and move the epigastric area.

　　口唇撮圆如管状，口唇前伸，舌两侧微卷放于口中间，有松开食道之意，气从喉出后，在口腔中形成一股中间气流，经撮圆的口唇呼出体外。

Shape of the lips/mouth: Pucker the lips into a round tube, extend the lips, and curl up the tongue towards the center (to relax the esophagus). The aspiration starts from the throat, forms an airflow and comes out through the rounded lips.

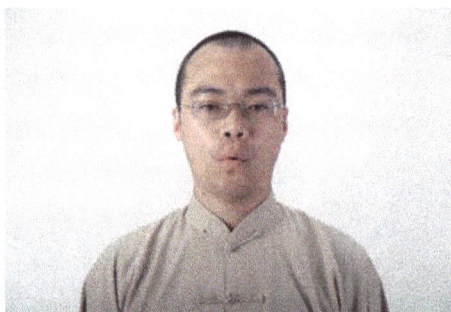

呼字口型图　　The lips/mouth shape of *Hu* sound

4. 呬字口型
4. The lips/mouth shape of *Hei* sound

呬字口型是人在幽怨烦闷自然发出"呬"（hei）的声音，声音比"呵"低沉。该口型自然带动整个胸部。发音为"hei"。

Hei is an involuntary sound when one feels sad and upset. It is lower and deeper than the *He* sound. The entire chest is involved in aspirating this sound.

唇齿微张，口腔略向两侧撑开，舌体略上台前送，下颌略下沉，有打开胸部之意，气从舌上与舌两侧缓缓而出。

Shape of the lips/mouth: Slightly open the lips and teeth, pull the mouth corners to both sides, extend the tongue body forward and slightly sink the lower jaw (to open up the chest). The aspiration comes out from the tongue and through both sides of the tongue.

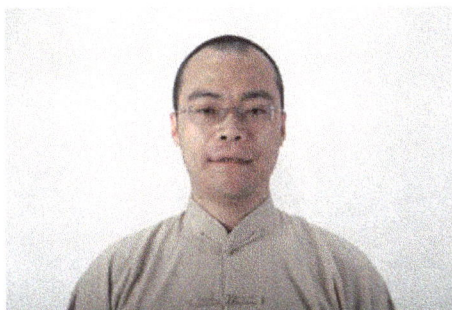

呬字口型图　　The lips/mouth shape of *Hei* sound

5. 吹字口型
5. The lips/mouth shape of *Chui* sound

吹字口型是人在寒冷、气机沉滞不通时会自然牙关用力的口型。该口型自然带动腰部。发吴音"吹",接近"ci"。

Chui is an involuntary sound when one feels cold or pain (due to qi stagnation). In *Wu* accent, it is similar to *Ci*. The waist area is involved in aspirating this sound.

唇齿只留一条缝,两腮向后收紧,嘴角后引,有打开腰部之意,两侧牙齿略用力,上下齿间留少许空隙,舌体微微上翘,舌尖与牙齿间留少许空隙,气出于上下齿与舌的狭缝间。

Shape of the lips/mouth: Almost close the lips and teeth, tighten the cheeks backward, and pull the mouth corners backward (to open up the waist area). Slightly use force on both sides of the teeth to allow some space between upper and lower teeth, curl up the tongue to leave some space between the tongue tip and teeth. The aspiration comes out through the space between upper, lower teeth and the tongue.

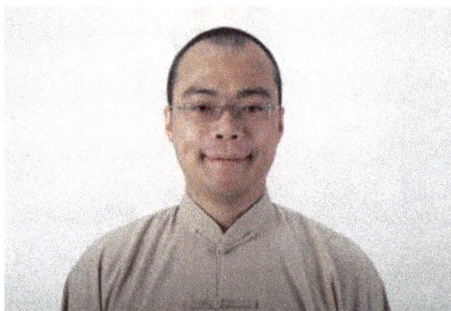

吹字口型图　The lips/mouth shape of *Chui* sound

6. 嘻字口型
6. The lips/mouth shape of *Xi* sound

嘻字口型是人在全身舒畅时发出"嘻"的声音。该口型自然带动整个躯干。发音为"xi"。

Xi is an involuntary sound when one feels comfortable and at ease. The torso is involved in aspirating this sound.

唇齿微开,嘴角略后引并上翘,舌尖放平并轻抵下齿中部,上下门牙对齐,气出于两边牙齿的缝隙。

Shape of the lips/mouth: Slightly open the lips and teeth, pull the mouth corners backward and curl up, keep the tongue tip flat and use the tongue tip to touch the middle part of the lower teeth, making the upper and lower front teeth touching each other. The aspiration comes out through the space between teeth on both sides.

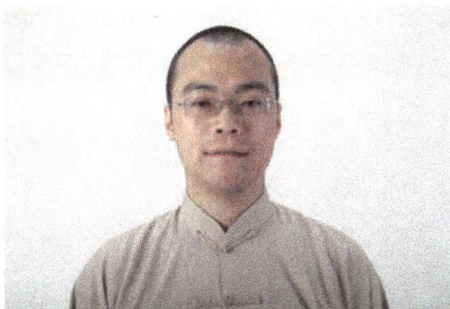

嘻字口型图　　The lips/mouth shape of *Xi* sound

呼吸操作
Respiration Method

普通人的呼吸方式多为胸式呼吸和顺腹式呼吸，在习练古音六字诀的过程中，随着身体不断的松柔，呼吸方式也会出现不同的变化，顺式呼吸将会扩大至腹部、命门、腰骶、夹脊等部位。随着丹田部位的主动性增加，呼吸形式将转化为逆式呼吸形式，随着内气的不断松透，慢慢将形成全身性的体呼吸。呼吸调整需要一定的基础，特别是意念要清净平淡，刻意调整呼吸容易出现呼吸的僵滞。对于初练者来讲，不建议进行呼吸操作，以自然呼吸为主。

In daily lives, ordinary people often use chest or abdominal breathing. Through practice of *Gu Yin Liu Zi Jue*, our body can become more soft and flexible. Over time, our breathing may also change. Abdominal breathing can gradually reach the abdomen, *Mingmen*[1], lumbosacral area and Jiaji[2] points. Along with increased activities in the Dantian area, one can start to conduct reverse abdominal breathing. Along with further exercise of internal qi, one can have the whole body breathing.

---

1. Mingmen literally means the gate of life, located between the kidneys, at the level of the second lumbar vertebrae.
2. A group of 34 points, 0.5 cun lateral to the lower border of the spinous processes from T_1 to L_5.

A tranquil peaceful mind is essential for breathing adjustment. Intentional breathing adjustment can impede respiration. Beginners should use natural breathing.

1. 顺式呼吸
1. Chest and abdominal breathing

顺式呼吸是以肺部为主带动的呼吸状态，人在站立时的自然呼吸形式一般是胸式呼吸；女子则胸式呼吸较多；胸式呼吸的特征为吸气时胸部鼓起，呼气时胸部回缩。

Chest breathing uses the middle area of the lungs by expanding and contracting the ribcage. When we stand, we usually use natural chest breathing. More commonly seen in women, chest breathing is characterized by chest bulging in inhalation and chest retraction in exhalation.

随着胸口的放松，腹式呼吸出现，气沉丹田，呼吸的深度加深。运动员、歌唱家大多是顺腹式呼吸；相比女子，男子的腹式呼吸易于出现。

Along with relaxation of the chest area, abdominal breathing can occur, coupled with qi sinking to Dantian area and a deeper breath. Most athletes and singers use abdominal breathing. Abdominal breathing is easier in men than women.

顺腹式呼吸是练功初期常用的呼吸方式，此时呼吸的时候胸骨不再上下前后活动，胸廓也基本不动，而是膈肌的上下运动。呼吸是肺的伸缩由原来的横向伸缩转变成为纵向伸缩。

Commonly used in early stage of qigong practice,

abdominal breathing is done by contracting the diaphragm rather than the movement of the breastbone and thoracic cage. Air enters the lungs and the belly expands during this type of breathing, i.e., a shift from the transverse movement of the lungs during chest breathing to longitudinal movement during abdominal breathing.

随着身体不断的松透，身体随呼吸起伏将不限于腹部，命门、腰骶、夹脊等部位都能随着呼吸进行起伏。

Over time, abdominal breathing can gradually reach the abdomen, *Mingmen*, lumbosacral area and Jiaji points.

2. 逆式呼吸
2. Reverse abdominal breathing

逆式呼吸是以丹田吐纳为主带动的呼吸状态，一般表现为逆腹式呼吸，是在内气产生后才能操作，需要老师指导，否则很容易出现气机僵滞等偏差症状。

Reverse abdominal breathing uses the exhaling and inhaling of the Dantian area. This depends on abundance of internal qi and instructions of the teacher. Otherwise, deviation symptoms such as impediment of qi activity may occur.

关于丹田的位置有两种说法：一则位于脐下三寸，二则位于脐内三寸，即躺着的脐下三寸。从机制上讲，逆式呼吸是丹田吐纳时带动膈肌的升降，从而带动肺容量改变，表现为逆腹式呼吸。其呼吸的动力源头在丹田：丹田纳气，腹部变小，膈肌下降，产生吸气现象；丹田吐气，腹部鼓出，膈肌上升，产生呼气现象；另外丹田呼吸时伴随身体气息的整体吐纳，不只局限于肺部。很多内气的锻炼都会用到丹田呼吸。专业训练歌唱家用的也是丹田之气。

There are two theories regarding the location of Dantian: one is located 3 cun below the umbilicus; the other is located 3 cun within the umbilicus i. e., 3cun beneath the umbilicus in a lying position. In terms of mechanism, reverse abdominal breathing uses the exhalation and inhalation of Dantian to contract the diaphragmatic muscle to change the lung capacity. Dantian is the power source of reverse abdominal breathing: the abdomen contracts inward during inhalation (the diaphragmatic muscle moves down) and relaxes outward during exhalation (the diaphragmatic muscle moves up). In addition, the whole body (not only the lungs) is involved in this breathing. This breathing method is often used in exercise of internal qi or training of professional singers.

随着心身松透后内气通达全身，整个身体会随着丹田吐纳而开合，出现全身皮毛与丹田呼吸相呼应形成的一种"开合呼吸""毫毛呼吸"，俗称"体呼吸"。此时随着丹田的一开一合，出现皮肤毛孔的一呼一吸，吸气时全身向丹田收合，毛孔也渐开；呼气时气从丹田向外扩散，毛孔也渐合。现在科学证明皮肤本身存在透气性。《庄子·大宗师》："古之真人，其寝不梦，其觉无忧，其食不甘，其息深深。圣人之息以踵，众人之息以喉。"是说圣人呼吸可以一直牵连到脚跟，而普通人一般只是局限在肺。

Over time, the whole body opens and closes with exhalation and inhalation of Dantian (known as the body respiration), manifesting as 'opening and closing respiration' or 'skin hair respiration' (the skin pores open when Dantian inhales and the skin pores close when Dantian exhales). Modern science has confirmed the breathability of the skin. The *Zhuang Zi Da Zong Shi* (Inner chapter 6 of Zhuangzi) states, 'The True Man of the antiquity slept without dreaming and woke without anxiety; he sought no sweetness in his food and he breathed as deeply as could be. The True Man breathes from his heels, where the common person breathes from his throat.'

随着身体进一步松透，口鼻呼吸就逐渐微细起来而近乎"若有若无，若存若止"，进入胎息状态。

Along with further relaxation of the body, the breathing through the mouth and nose gradually becomes indistinct and enters the fetal (embryonic) breathing state.

基本操作
Basic Movements

1. 握固
1. *Wo Gu* (Firm Grasping)

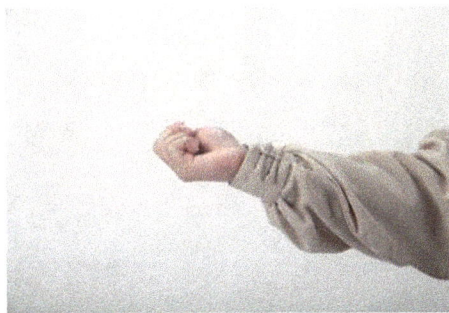

握固示意图　　*Wo Gu* (Firm Grasping)

握固方法为大拇指掐在其他三个手指的掌指横纹上，指尖抵环指根部，以余四指握大拇指成拳，《道枢·众妙篇》："握固者何也？吾以左右拇指掐其三指之文，或以四指总握其拇。"《诸病源候论》说："两手各自以四指把手拇指。"握固有助于安魂定神，收摄精气。

This method means to use the thumb to pinch the transverse crease of the three fingers, and touch the base of the ring finger with the tip of the thumb and make a fist by grasping the thumb with the other four fingers. The *Dao Shu Zhong Miao Pian* (One chapter in the Pivot of Dao) states, 'What is firm grasping? It's a fist made by using the thumb to pinch the transverse crease of the three fingers or placing the thumb under the other four fingers'. The *Zhu Bing Yuan Hou Lun* (Treatise on the Origins and Manifestations of Various Diseases) states, 'for both hands, place the thumb under the other four fingers'. Firm grasping can help to calm the mind and hold essential qi.

2. 立掌
2. *Li Zhang* (Standing Palm)

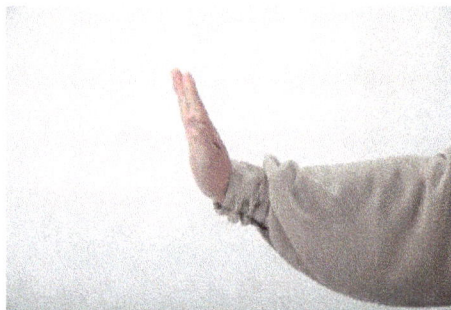

立掌示意图　*Li Zhang* (Standing Palm)

立掌，又称"坐腕"。五指稍分开，指微屈不直，掌心微内凹，指中节有向手背之意，意劲贯注指肚，腕关节柔而软，掌根沉住。

Standing palm, also known as sitting wrist, means to slightly separate and flex the five fingers, making the palms slightly face inward and middle knuckles face toward the dorsa of the hands. This can help to concentrate mental focus on the finger pad, enable the wrist joint to be soft and flexible and the base of the palm more stable.

3. 提肛
3. *Ti Gang* (Lifting up the Anus)

提肛，又称"撮谷道"，轻轻地使肛门周围的肌肉及软组织收缩，然后放松，一收一松，反复进行，见于孙思邈的养生十三法。据传乾隆皇帝能活到89岁高龄，成为我国历代皇帝中的最高寿者，这与他几十年如一日地坚持"撮谷道"不无关系。"撮谷道"可以使整个盆腔肌肉特别是骶髂肌得到运动锻炼，是内功锻炼的入门方法。需要注意的是收的时候不可用力屏，只需轻轻有点感觉就行。

Lifting up the anus (also known as Cuo Gu Dao in Chinese) means to gently contract and relax the muscles and soft tissue around the anus. This was recorded in the 13 health cultivation methods by Sun Si-miao. As the story goes, the Qianlong Emperor of the Manchu-led Qing Dynasty became the most longevity emperor in Chinese history because he had been practicing lifting up the anus every day. Lifting up the anus can exercise the pelvic cavity muscles, especially the sacroiliac muscle, which serves as an introduction to internal exercise.

Caution: Do not use too much force during contraction (a sense of contraction is enough).

4. 站桩

4. *Zhan Zhuang* (Standing Like a Post)

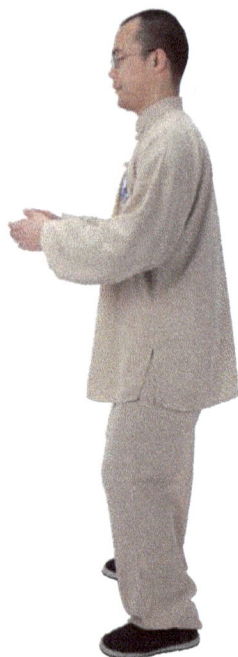

站桩示意图　*Zhan Zhuang*

古音六字诀采用站立姿势，站姿的好坏直接影响锻炼的效果。总的来讲，站桩位时要做到沉肩坠肘、伸腰沉胯、两腿含劲、含胸拔背、虚灵顶劲。

The *Gu Yin Liu Zi Jue* uses the standing posture. A good standing posture will bring about good effect. General requirements of *Zhan Zhuang* include: Sink the shoulders and drop the elbows, straighten the low back, relax the hip joints, use force on the legs, tuck in the chest and pull up the back and pull up your Baihui (DU 20)[1] point on the top of your head.

––––––––––––

1. At the junction of a line connecting the apices of the ears (in the middle).

沉肩坠肘是上身放松，气机松沉的表现，初练者由于腰胯相对虚弱，习惯借助上身肩背力量出现抗肩，提肘的现象。要做到沉肩坠肘不仅在主观上要放松肢体，也需要身体放松后内气条达的自然舒展力。其感觉犹如醉汉的胳膊，松软但是很沉抬不起的感觉，也有"棉里裹铁"的说法。

It's important to relax the shoulders and elbows and let them hang down for beginners. At first, beginners tend to use the force of the upper body, especially the shoulder and back, manifesting as raising the shoulder or elbow. Sinking the shoulders and dropping the elbows is not only about relaxing the arms but also free flow of internal qi. The vivid description goes that a drunken man cannot lift his arms although his arms feel soft and relaxed, which is also known as 'iron wrapped in a piece of cotton'.

当气沉丹田时自然会出现含胸的现象，此时人的胸骨放松下垂，两肩如含，但也要避免刻意扣胸。当气沉丹田后将会自然出现顺腹式呼吸。

The chest is slightly reserved inward when qi sinks to Dantian. This can often be followed by abdominal breathing. However, it's important not to tuck in the chest intentionally.

腰是身体活动的中枢，主宰身体四肢的运动，伸腰讲的是腰的伸展性，也就是老祖宗说的腰板要挺直。现代的人由于各种生活习惯，体力劳动缺失，导致腰部力气的虚弱，往往没法伸展腰部，伸腰的表现为人的腰部的生理曲度随着伸腰能够相对变直，出现命门往后走的现象。在临床上很多腰不好的人就是因为腰力不够，腰板没法挺起来，在长时间的坐姿、站姿，在外力下导致腰部承受不了出现腰椎滑脱、椎间盘突出等。

The waist is the commander of the whole body. Only after

you are able to straighten up the low back will the two legs have strength and the lower body be stable. In modern society, we often feel weakness in the low back due to lack of physical labor. As a result, many people may develop lumbar spondylolisthesis or lumbar intervertebral disc herniation from long-time sitting, standing or external force.

胯的操作需要一定的基础，历来有传腰不传胯的说法。普通人习惯用身体前侧的力量，在练功中常常会出现挺胯的现象，但在收胯的时候又会出现翘臀的现象。其关键就是胯没有沉下去，也就是尾间没有下垂。当胯沉好后还要敛臀提肛，像夹着尾巴的感觉。胯的操作需要腰部和骶髂关节甚至尾骨的放松，操作上比较难，没有松静基础的人很难做到。

It's not easy to relax the hip joints. Since we tend to use more force from the front of our body, beginners often present with hip extension. However, when they try to retract the hip joint, they may lift the buttocks. It's essential to drop the hip joint or the coccyx, tuck the buttocks in and lift up the anus, just like holding the tail between the legs. To relax the hip joint, you need to relax the waist, sacroiliac joint and tail bone. As a result, it takes some time to practice.

站桩中一旦做到沉胯，腿上就会感觉到非常的吃力，此时就是锻炼两腿的劲，也就是平时说的脚劲，有"入地三尺"的说法。经过一段时间的锻炼，腿的前后内外侧的肌肉韧带都能得到控制，练古音六字诀时两脚的位置要略宽于肩部。

Once the hip joints are relaxed, it's time to build up strength of the legs, i.e., the strength of the feet (the root is three feet into the floor). You need to exercise the anterior, posterior, medial and lateral muscles and ligaments of the legs for some time. During exercise of *Gu Yin Liu Zi Jue*, keep a wider feet distance than the shoulders.

拔背是将脊柱伸展开，是伸腰的进一步伸展，属于背部夹脊部位的伸展，其基础是脚上要有根劲，腰部的充分松展，内气开始往上通达，敛气入脊，出现背部拔伸的现象。不可勉强上拔，把气提上来。拔背后胸椎的生理曲度也会相对变直。

Further to straighten up the low back, pulling up the back means to stretch the spine or Jiaji points. To do this, you need to have root in the feet and a fully relaxed waist to allow internal qi enters the spine. Do not force yourself to pull up the back; otherwise, the physiological curve of the thoracic vertebrae will also straighten up.

有了腰部和背部的伸展基础后，颈部的椎体间也会出现伸展，此时气敛入颈椎，整个脊柱松透，内气条达，脊柱内的脊髓和神经都能够得到濡养，体质出现质的改善。由于是松透后内气自然撑顶的原因，不是勉强伸展，所以感觉上是虚灵的。

After the waist and back are straightened, cervical vertebra can also be stretched. With relaxation of the spine, internal qi can nourish the spinal cord and nerves and thus improve one's body constitution. Since this whole process is done naturally inside the body, you'll feel empty and free.

此一段站桩是古音六字诀的基础站姿，也是练功的重要部分，其本身也需要几年以上的锻炼才能逐步到位。

As a basic and essential part of *Gu Yin Liu Zi Jue, Zhan Zhuang* may take years of practice.

具 体 操 作

Individual Movements

起势　松静三调

Starting posture (Three Regulations to be Relaxed and Tranquil)

1. 调心

1. Regulation of the mind

调整到轻松愉快的情绪状态中，感受自身气机的轻松安宁。

This aims to achieve a light-hearted, peaceful and tranquil state.

2. 调身

2. Regulation of the body

松静站立，两脚自然分开，略
比肩宽，两膝微曲。重心落在脚
跟，十个脚趾微扣，脚底心内含。
两手自然垂抱于小腹前。目平视。

Stand in relaxation and tranquil
and separate the feet to shoulder-width
(or wider) apart. Slightly bend the
knee and place the body weight on the
heels. Slightly turn the toes downward
and tuck in the soles. Drop the hands
naturally in front of the abdomen and
look straight ahead.

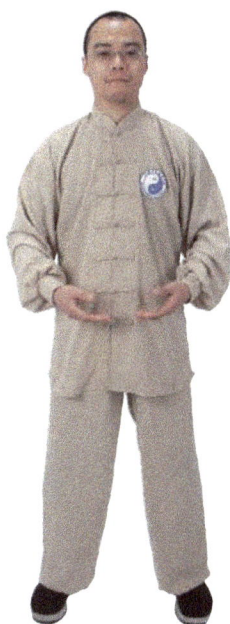

起势图 1-1　Starting posture 1-1

3. 调息

3. Regulation of the breathing

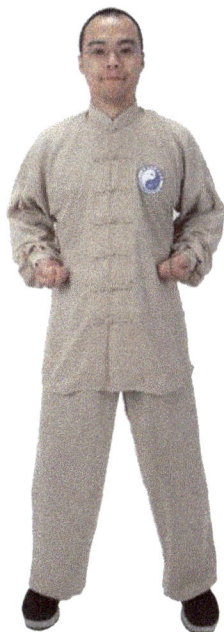

吸气，两手自腹前上提成握
固，收至两腰旁；同时提肛。

Breathe in (inhale): Place the thumb
under the other four fingers and lift the
hands above the hip bones, and lift up the
anus.

起势图 1-2　Starting posture 1-2

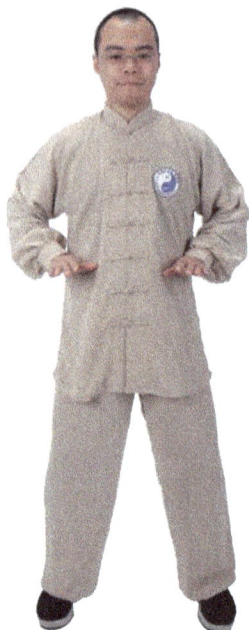

呼气，双拳放开，翻掌。

Breathe out (exhale): Release the fists, turn the palms.

起势图 1-3　Starting posture 1-3

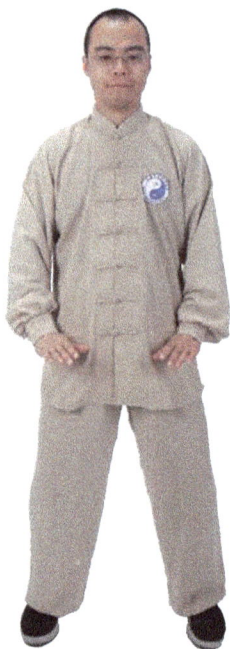

下按至胯前，胸骨向下松，腹部放松。感觉犹如人忙完事情后，心头的一块石头落了下来的感觉。

Press the palms downward to the hip bones, relax the breast bone and abdomen. After this, one feels relieved or a load off the mind.

起势图 1-4　Starting posture 1-4

重复3次。

Repeat 3 times.

第一势　肝若嘘时目瞪睛
Movement # 1　The *Xu* sound

犹如紧张时自然发出的声音，发音为"xu"。

A natural vibration of sound *(Xu)* when you are nervous.

动作一：

Step # 1:

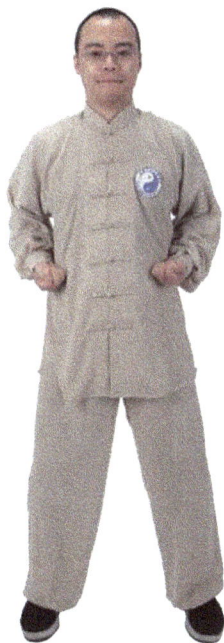

两手自腹前上提成握固，收至两腰旁，同时吸气，提肛。

Place the thumb under the other four fingers and lift the hands above the hip bones. At the same time, inhale and lift up the anus.

图 1-1　Fig 1-1

动作二：

Step # 2:

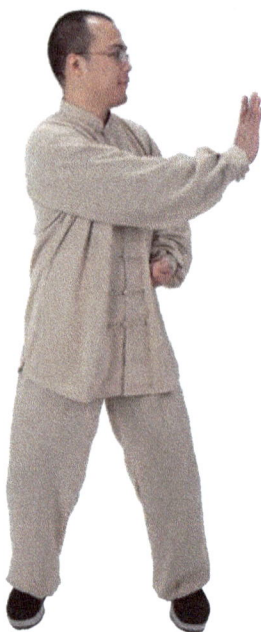

右腿保持不动，右胯撑开，右侧大脚趾抓地，腰以下尽量不动，腰部左转，顺势右手从腰部成掌向左侧推出；同时发"嘘"字音，眼睛瞪大。

Keep the right leg still, extend the right hip to grasp the floor with the great toe of the right feet. Turn the low back (try not to move the lower body) to left, extend the right palm towards the left and aspirate the syllable of *Xu* and make the eyes wide open.

图 1-2　Fig 1-2

动作三：

Step # 3:

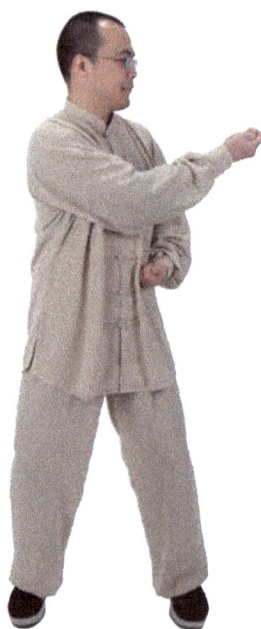

手掌外旋，五指向下，收成握固状。

Turn the palm outward and five fingers downward. place the thumb under the other four fingers.

图 1-3　Fig 1-3

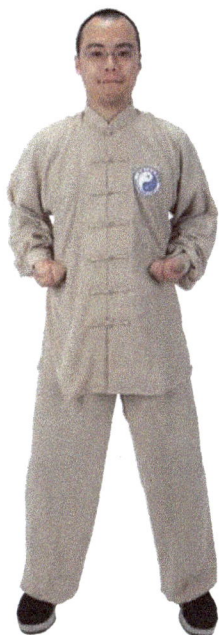

腰回旋，同时手收回至腰两侧，拳心向上；同时吸气。

Rotate the low back, and retract the hands above the hip bones, make the fists upward and inhale.

图 1-4　Fig 1-4

动作四：
Step # 4:

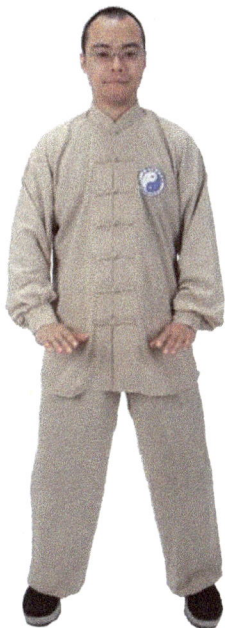

双拳放开，翻掌下按至胯前，松静站立；同时呼气。

Release the fists, turn and press the palms downward to the hip bones, stand in relaxation and tranquil and exhale.

图 1-5　Fig 1-5

重复6次。

Repeat 6 times.

［动作要点］撑开时腰部尽量不动，胯部撑开，使得足厥阴肝经得到牵拉。胁肋至背部张开，牵拉到夹脊部位。

[Key Principles]

◇ Try not to move the low back when opening up the hip joints.

◇ To pull the liver meridian of foot-Jueyin, rib area, back, and Jiaji points.

第二势　心呵顶上连叉手
Movement # 2　The *He* sound

犹如开心时自然发出的笑声，发音为吴音的"喝"。接近"he""ha"。

A natural vibration of laughter sound (*He* or *Ha*) when you are happy.

动作一：

Step # 1:

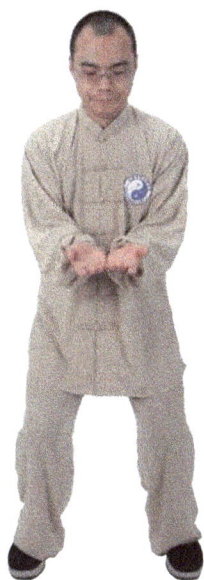

两手自腹前掌心朝上，十指向前，小指相靠。

Place the hands in front of the abdomen and turn the palms upward, making the ten fingers forward and two little fingers close to each other.

图 2-1   Fig 2-1

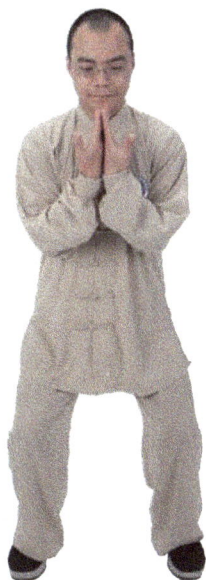

以尺侧小指引领上提至胸前，成十指向上，掌背相靠；同时吸气、提肛。

Guide and lift the hands to the level of chest using the ulnar side of the little finger, making the ten fingers upward and the dorsa of the hands close to each other. Simultaneously, inhale and lift up the anus.

图 2-2   Fig 2-2

动作二：

Step # 2:

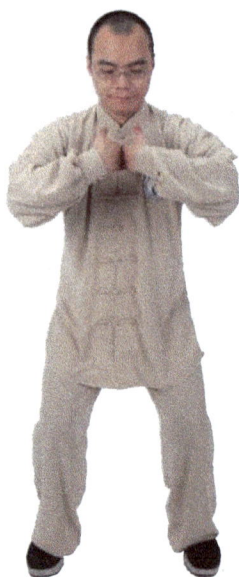

掌背相靠，十指环转向内。

Place the dorsa of the hands together and turn the ten fingers inward.

图 2-3　Fig 2-3

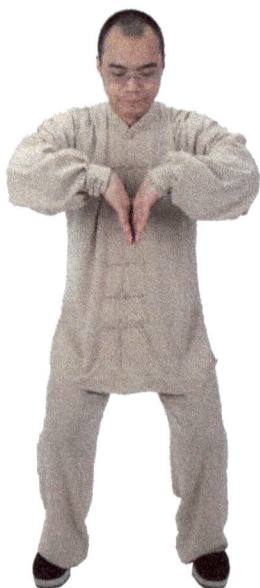

十指向下。

Turn the ten fingers downward.

图 2-4　Fig 2-4

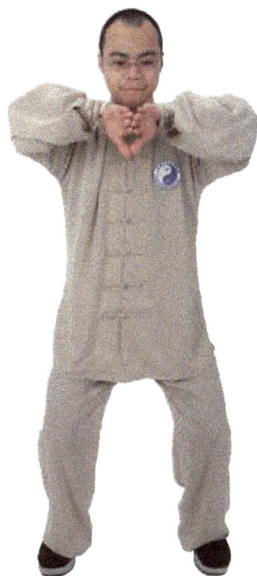

十指向外。

Turn the ten fingers outward.

图 2-5　Fig 2-5

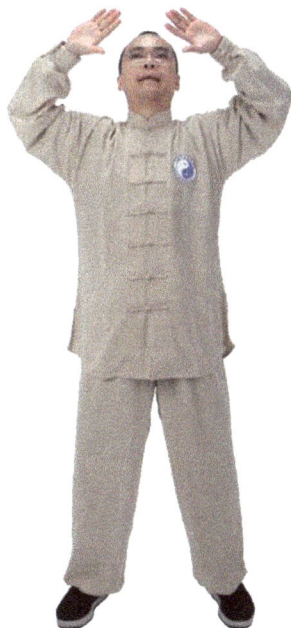

然后扩胸，以尺侧小指引领，
双手打开至头两侧，尺侧外旋；
同时发"呵"字音。

Expand the chest, guide and open the hands using the ulnar side of the little finger to both sides of the head. Turn the ulnar side outward and aspirate the syllabus of 'He'.

图 2-6　Fig 2-6

动作三：

Step # 3:

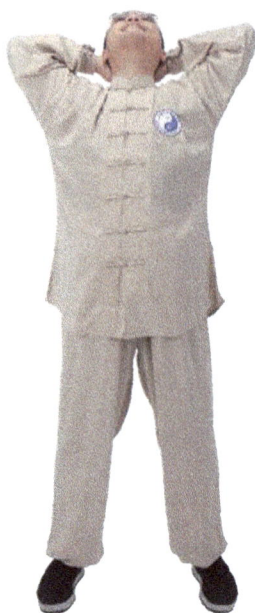

正面　front

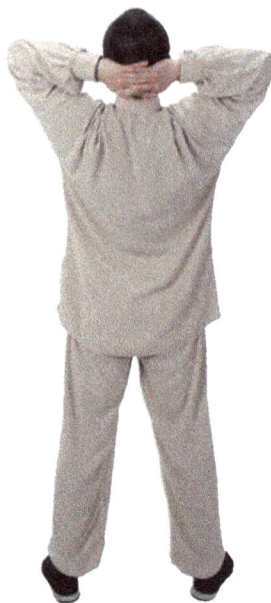

背面　back

图 2-7　Fig 2-7

双手手指交叉于头后，头颈后仰使胸廓进一步打开；同时吸气。

Place the hands with crossed fingers on the occiput, extend the head and neck to further expand the chest and inhale.

动作四：
Step # 4:

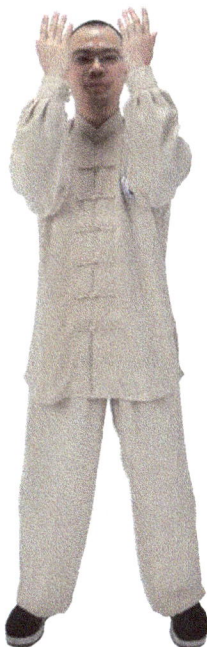

两手松开，尺侧内旋，掌心
向内，回至面前；同时呼气。

Release the hands, turn ulnar
side and palms of the hands inward,
place the hands in front of the face,
and exhale.

图 2-8   Fig 2-8

动作五：
Step # 5:

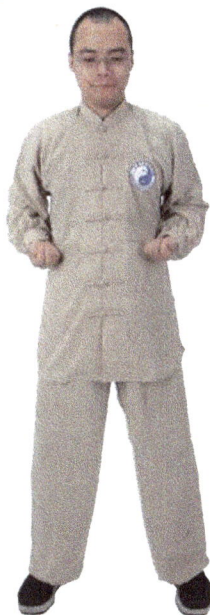

双手自面前下落收回至腰两
侧，握固，拳心向上；同时吸气。

Drop the hands to both sides of
the hip bone, turn the palms downward,
place the thumb under the other four
fingers, make the fists upward and
inhale.

图 2-9   Fig 2-9

动作六：

Step # 6:

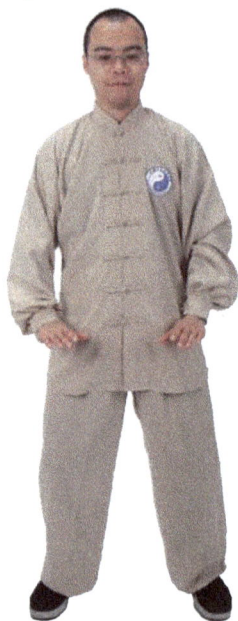

双拳放开，翻掌下按至胯前，松静站立；同时呼气。

Release the fists, turn and press the palms down to the hipbone, stand in relaxation and tranquil and exhale.

图 2-10　Fig 2-10

重复6次。

Repeat 6 times.

[动作要点] 两手动作以手少阴心经为引导，感觉手部尺侧有牵拉感。打开至头两侧时扩胸，十指交叉在项后时，颈项后仰，使得胸廓进一步扩张，同时可以想象自己躺在草地上晒太阳的感觉。回收时同样用尺侧为引导。

[Key Principles]

◇ Use the heart meridian of hand-Shaoyin to guide movements of the hands and have a pulling sensation on ulnar sides of the hands.

◇ Expand the chest when opening the hands to both sides of the head and further expand the chest by extending the neck when placing the hands with crossed fingers on the occiput. At the same time, imagine you are lying on the grass in sunlight.

◇ Use the ulnar side of the heads to guide retraction of the hands.

第三势　脾病呼时须撮口
Movement # 3　The *Hu* sound

犹如吃饱时自然发出的声音,发音为"hu"。

A natural vibration of laughter sound (*He* or *Ha*) when your stomach is full.

动作一:

Step # 1:

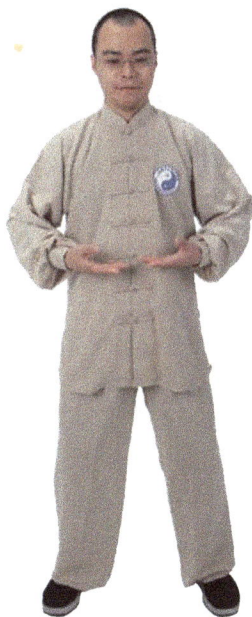

两手自腹前掌心朝上,十指相对,上提至腹前;同时吸气、提肛。

Place the hands in front of the abdomen, make the palms upward and ten fingers facing each other and lift the hands to the level of the chest, inhale and lift up the anus.

图 3-1　Fig 3-1

动作二:

Step # 2:

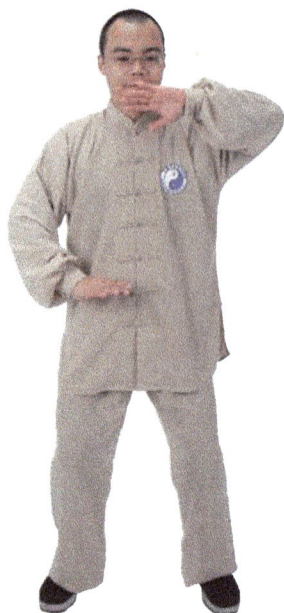

两手翻掌向下，左手掌心外翻，左胁上拔。

Turn the palms downward. Then turn the left palm outward, and pull up the left rib area.

图 3–2　Fig 3–2

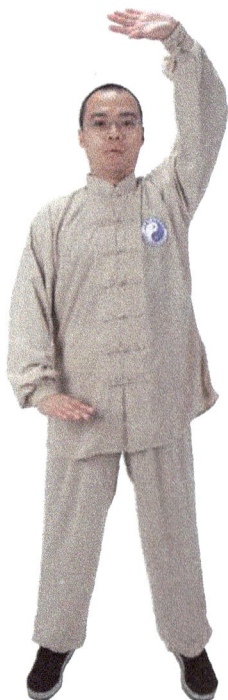

左手自体前反托向上，掌心朝上；右掌下按至右腿侧，踮脚站立；同时发"呼"字音。

Lift the left hand from the front of the body (palm upward). Turn the right palm and press down to the lateral side of the leg, stand on tiptoe and aspirate the syllabus of *Hu*.

图 3–3　Fig 3–3

动作三：

Step # 3:

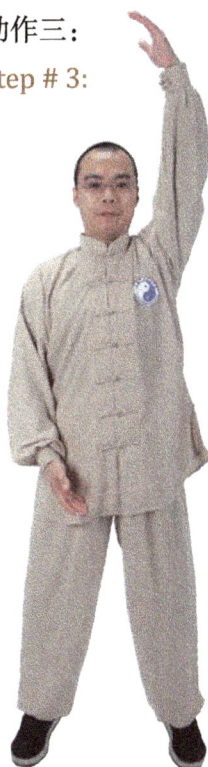

两手翻掌,掌心相对。

Turn the palms to face each other.

图 3-4　Fig 3-4

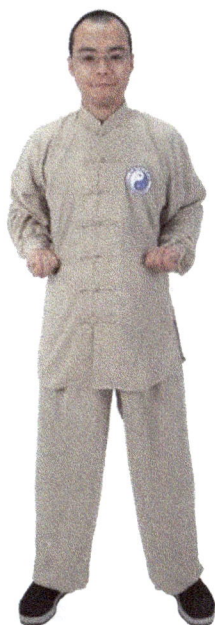

收回至腰两侧、握固,拳心向上,两脚落下;同时吸气。

Retract the palms to both sides of the waist, place the thumb under the other four fingers, turn the fists upward, drop the feet and inhale.

图 3-5　Fig 3-5

动作四：

Step # 4:

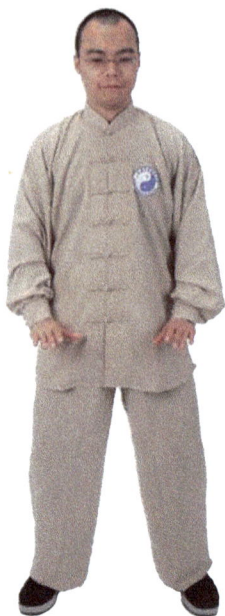

双拳放开，翻掌下按至胯前，松静站立；同时呼气。

Release the fists, turn the palms and press down to the front of the hip bone, stand in relaxation and tranquil and exhale.

图 3–6　Fig 3–6

左右各3次；重复6次。

Perform 3 times on each side and repeat 6 times.

［动作要点］一伸一降时以前面与侧面的躯体作为拔伸，手部放松自然伸展，踮脚时以第一、第二脚趾用力为主，刺激脾经与胃经。

[Key Principles]

◇ Pull and extend using the front and bilateral sides of the body during ascent and descent.

◇ Relax and extend the hands.

◇ Place the body weight on the great and second toes when standing on tiptoe to stimulate the spleen and stomach meridians[1].

_____

1. The spleen meridian starts from the medial side of the great toe and the stomach meridian terminates at the lateral side of the second toe.

第四势 肺和咽气手双擎
Movement # 4   The *Hei* sound

犹如幽怨烦闷时自然发出的声音,发音为 "hei"。

A natural vibration of *hei* when you feel sad and upset

动作一:

Step # 1:

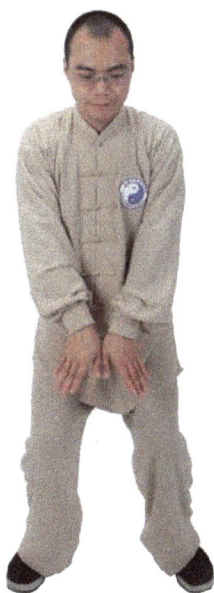

两手自腹前掌心朝内, 两大拇指相靠,十指向下。

Place the hands in front of the abdomen, making the thumbs touch each other and ten fingers downward.

图 4-1   Fig 4-1

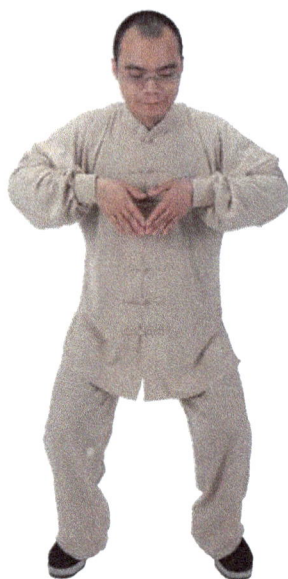

上提至胸前，掌心朝内，虎口相对；同时吸气、提肛。

Lift the hands to the level of chest, turn the palms inward and make the *Hukou* (space between the thumb and index finger) areas facing each other, inhale and lift up the anus.

图 4-2   Fig 4-2

动作二：

Step # 2:

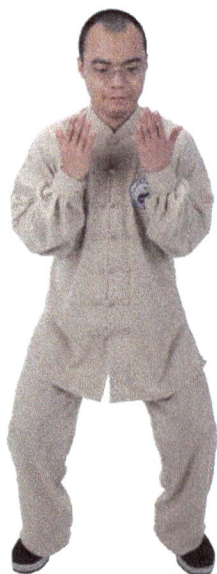

双手掌心朝内，指尖转向上。

Turn the palms inward, making the fingertips upward.

图 4-3   Fig 4-3

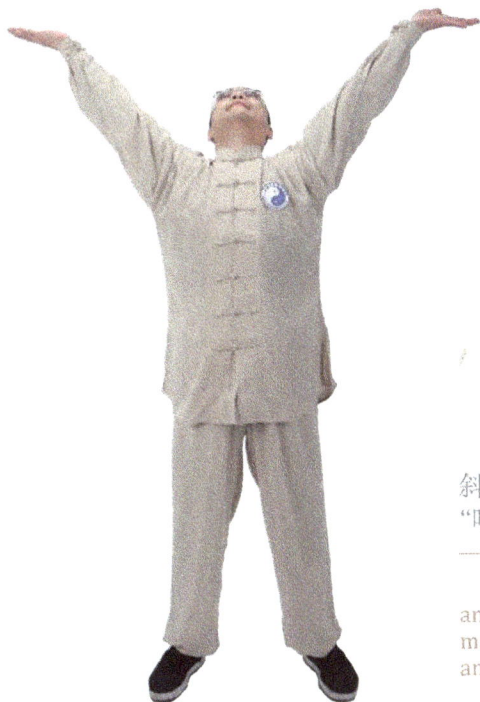

双手转为掌心朝上，向两侧斜上方托举，十指朝外；同时发"呬"字音。

Then turn the palms upward and lift the hands upward obliquely, make the ten fingers facing outward and aspirate the syllabus of *hei*.

图 4–4　Fig 4–4

动作三：

Step # 3:

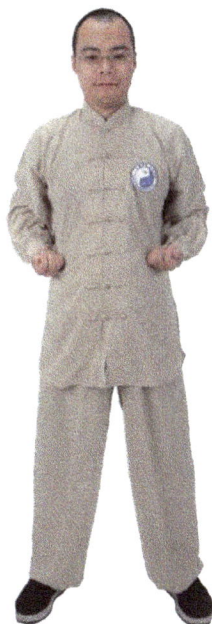

两手自胸前收回至腰两侧，握固，拳心向上；同时吸气。

Retract the hands from the chest to both sides of the waist, place the thumb under the other four fingers, turn the fists upward and inhale.

图 4–5　Fig 4–5

动作四:

Step # 4:

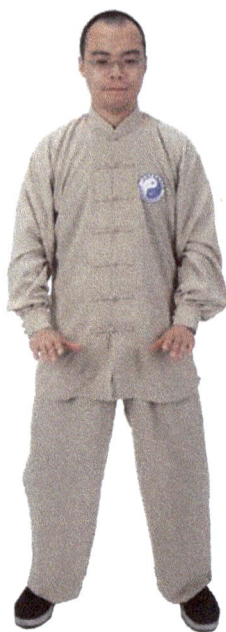

双拳放开，翻掌下按至胯前，
松静站立；同时呼气。

Release the fists, turn the palms
and press down to the front of the
hip bone, stand in relaxation and
tranquil and exhale.

图 4–6　Fig 4–6

重复6次。

Repeat 6 times.

［动作要点］两手以手太阴肺经为引导，手部桡侧有牵拉感，两手内合至上托时路线呈半圆形，上托时虎口张开，两肩向外上展开，扩张胸部。

[Key Principles]

◇ Use the lung meridian of hand-Taiyin to guide the hands and have a pulling sensation on radial sides of the hand.

◇ Keep a semicircular arc when turning the hands inward and lifting up the hands. During hands lifting, remember to open the *Hukou* areas, unfold the shoulder outward and upward to expand the chest.

第五势　肾吹抱取膝头平
Movement # 5　The *Chui* sound

犹如疼痛、寒冷时发出的声音，发音为吴音的"吹"，接近"ci"。

A natural vibration of *Chui* when you feel pain or cold.

动作一：

Step # 1:

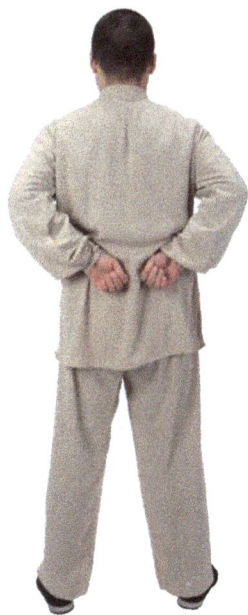

两手自腰后握固，拳背贴腰，拳眼相对，上提至两肾处；同时吸气、提肛。

Place the thumb under the other four fingers from behind the waist, make the dorsa of the fists touching the waist and the eyes of the fists (area between the thumb and index finger) facing each other, lift the hands to the location of kidneys, and inhale and lift up the anus.

图 5-1　Fig 5-1

动作二：
Step # 2:

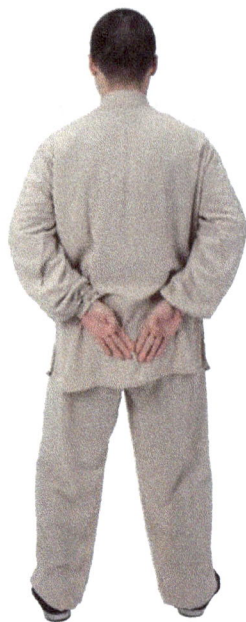

两拳松开成掌。

Release the fists.

图 5-2　Fig 5-2

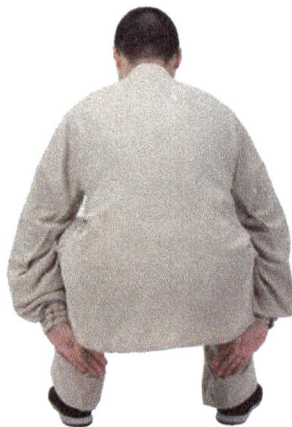

掌背沿大腿后侧下滑至足跟，
同时两腿下蹲；同时发"吹"字音。

Drop the palms down to the heels
along the posterior aspect of the thigh,
squat down and aspirate the syllabus of
Chui.

图 5-3　Fig 5-3

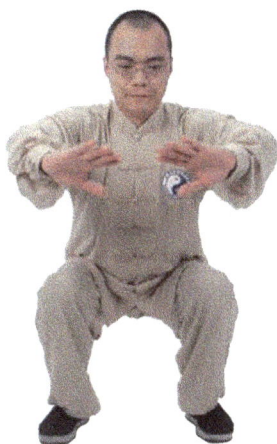

然后直腰成马步，两手顺势撑圆上提至平，掌心朝外拇指向下。

Then straighten the low back to a horse stance, make a circle with the hands and lift the hands to the level of the chest (palms outward, thumbs downward).

图 5-4　Fig 5-4

动作三：
Step # 3:

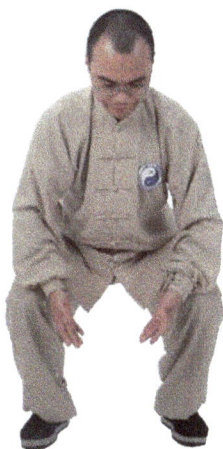

裹胯收臀，将上身撑起，两肘下落，顺势旋掌至掌心朝上。

Squeeze the hip, keep the buttocks tucked in, hold the upper body up, drop the elbows and turn the fists upward.

图 5-5　Fig 5-5

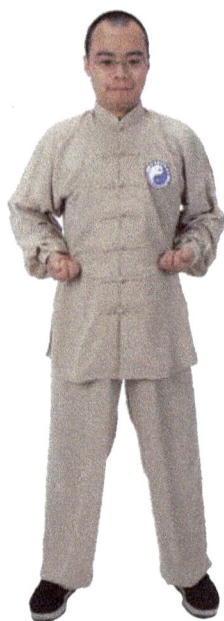

两手收回至腰两侧，握固，拳心向上；同时吸气。

Retract the hands to both sides of the waist, place the thumb under the other four fingers, keep the fists upward and inhale.

图 5-6　Fig 5-6

动作四：
Step # 4:

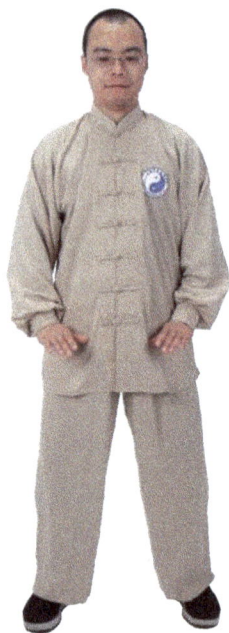

双拳放开、翻掌下按至胯前，松静站立；同时呼气。

Release the fists, turn the palms and press down to the front of the hip bone, stand in relaxation and tranquil and exhale.

图 5-7　Fig 5-7

重复6次。

Repeat 6 times.

[动作要点] 下蹲高度根据个人体质因人而异，不需强求。起身时要用胯的开合力量，将上身撑起，不用大腿的肌肉力量，这直接关系到锻炼的效果。

[Key Principles]

◇ Do not force yourself to squat down too much and do not feel bad if you cannot do as others.

◇ Use the opening and closing of the hip (instead of the thigh muscle) to help you stand up, since this is directly associated with the exercise effect.

第六势　三焦客热卧嘻宁
Movement # 6　The *Xi* sound

犹如全身舒畅时面带微笑发出"xi"的声音。

A natural vibration of Xi when you feel comfortable and smile.

动作一：

Step # 1:

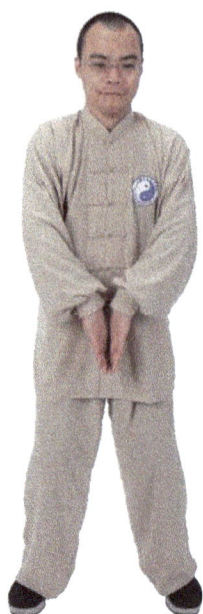

两手自腹前掌心朝外，掌背相靠，十指向下。

Place the hands in front of the abdomen with the palms outward, dorsa of the palms touching each other and ten fingers downward.

图 6-1   Fig 6-1

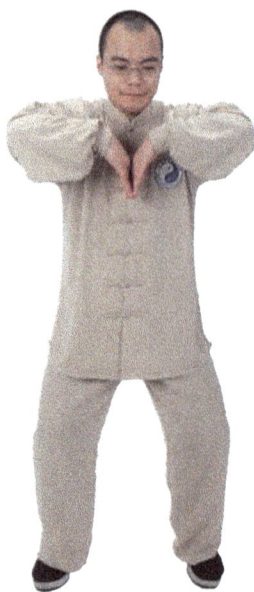

上提至胸前；同时吸气、提肛。

Lift the hands to the level of the chest, and inhale and lift up the anus.

图 6-2   Fig 6-2

动作二：

Step # 2:

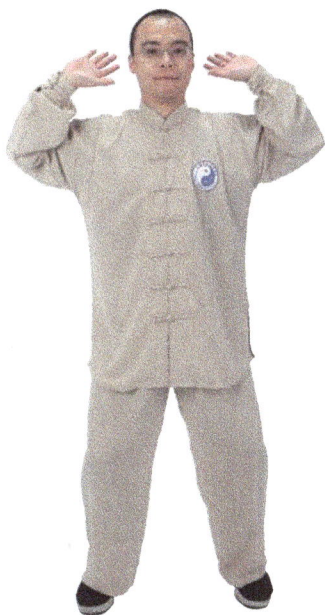

两手沿颈部两侧上提至耳
后，翻掌。

Lift the hands to the area behind
the ears along both sides of the neck,
turn the palms.

图 6-3　　Fig 6-3

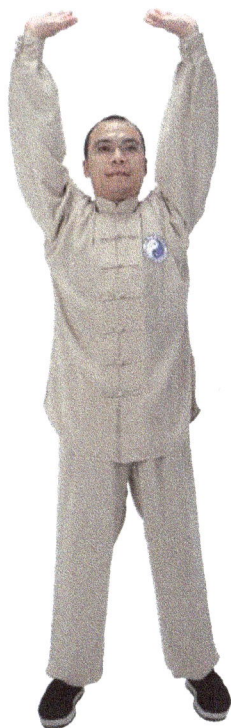

拔背，双手上托，掌心朝上，
虎口相对；同时发"嘻"字音。

pull the back, hold the hands
up (palms upward and Hukou areas
facing each other) and aspirate the
syllabus of *Xi*

图 6-4　　Fig 6-4

动作三：

Step # 3:

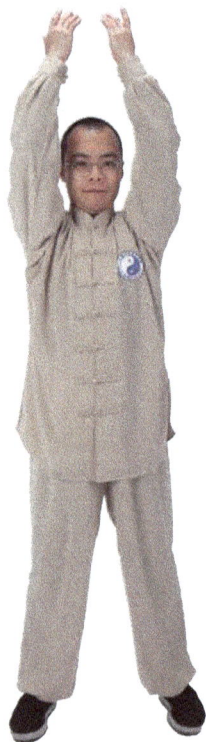

两掌旋转至面前下落。

Turn and drop the palms to the front of the face.

图 6-5   Fig 6-5

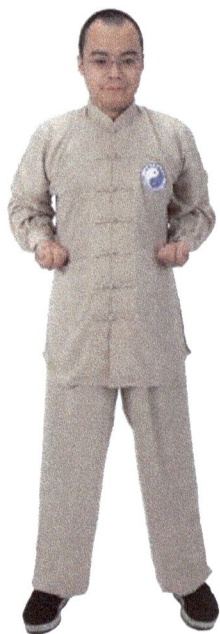

收回至腰两侧，握固，拳心向上；同时吸气。

Drop the hands to both sides of the waist, place the thumb under the other four fingers.with palms upward and inhale.

图 6-6   Fig 6-6

动作四：

Step # 4:

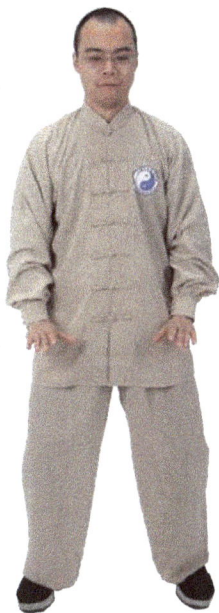

双拳放开，翻掌下按至胯前，松静站立；同时呼气。

Release the fists, turn the palms and press down to the front of the hip bone, stand in relaxation and tranquil and exhale.

图 6-7　Fig 6-7

重复6次。

Repeat 6 times.

［动作要点］两手手背相靠牵拉三焦经，上提时用躯体带动两手，上撑时为躯体上下开合，带动两手向上松柔舒展，不用手勉强上撑。下落时可用手指轻轻滑过皮肤，用自身手上的气感放松肌肤。

[Key Principles]

◇ To let dorsa of the hands touch each other to pull the Sanjiao meridian.

◇ Use the body to lift the hands (do not use the force of the hands). When dropping the hands, gently touch the skin with fingers (to relax the skin with qi sensation in the hands).

收势　静养丹田
Concluding posture　nourish the *Dantian*

1. 气归丹田
1. Return qi to *Dantian*

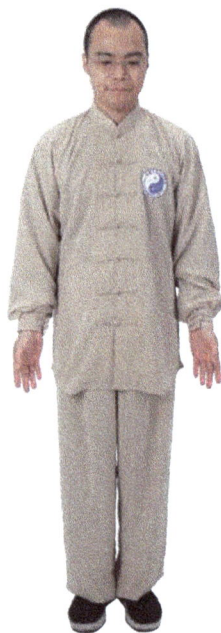

收势图 1-1　Concluding posture 1-1

左脚收回，两脚并拢。

Retract the left foot and place the feet together.

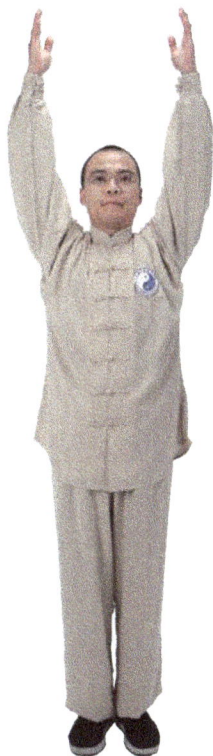

吸气，两手掌心向上，从体侧上举至头。

Inhale, turn the palms upward and lift the hands above the vertex from both sides of the body.

收势图 1-2　Concluding posture 1-2

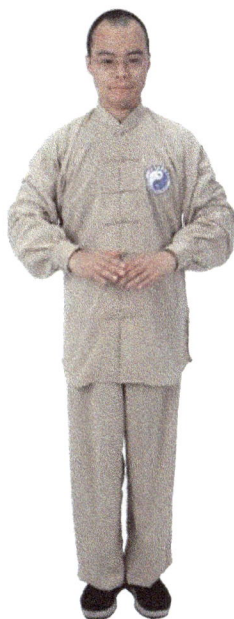

呼气，两手自体前下落至丹田处。

Exhale and drop the hands to Dantian from both sides of the body.

收势图 1-3　Concluding posture 1-3

重复3次。

Repeat 3 times.

2. 按摩丹田

2. Massage *Dantian*

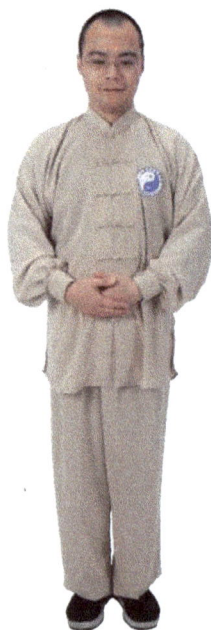

收势图 1–4　Concluding posture 1–4

男士左手在内，女士右手在内。顺时针按揉6次，再逆时针按揉6次。静养片刻。

Place the left hand beneath the right hand for men and the right hand beneath the left hand for women. Perform 6 times of clockwise pressing and kneading and 6 times of counterclockwise pressing and kneading. Keep still for a while.

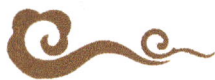

Application

应用

古 代 应 用

Ancient application

六字诀正式见于《养性延命录》的记载，"凡人之息，一呼一吸，原有此数。欲为长息吐气之法，时寒可吹，时温可呼。吹以去热，呼以去风，唏以去烦，呵以下气，嘘以散滞，呬以解极……若患者依此法，皆须恭敬，用心为之，无有不差，此即愈病长生要旨也。"文中所述六字气主治病症，以实证居多。即多于泻实而少于补虚。

The six healing sounds were officially recorded in the *Yang Xing Yan Ming Lu* (Records on Nourishing Character & Prolonging Life) written by Tao Hong-jing in the Southern and Northern Dynasties (420–589). The text states, '... One has only one way for inhalation but six for exhalation. *Chui* removes pathogenic cold or heat, *Hu* dissipates pathogenic wind and warmth, *Xi* relieves worries, *He* causes qi to descend, *Xu* resolves stagnation and *hei* improves exhaustion ... Practice these breathing exercises can help to recover from diseases and achieve longevity'. According to these descriptions, six sounds are more commonly indicated for excessive syndrome instead of deficiency syndrome, i.e., they are more used to reduce excess than reinforce deficiency.

历史上对于六字诀的功效应用描述较多，其中以胡愔所撰的《黄庭内景五脏六腑补泻图》中关于六字诀治疗应用的记载较为详尽，为后世所认可。

Historically there are numerous descriptions regarding

the functions of six healing sounds. The description recorded in the *Huang Ting Nei Jing Wu Zang Liu Fu Bu Xie Tu* (Illustrations of Reinforcing and Reducing Five-Zang and Six-Fu Organs, Scripture on the Internal View of the Yellow Court) by Hu Yin is well accepted by the later generations.

1. 嘘的应用
1. The *Xu* sound

"肝之有疾当用嘘。嘘者肝之气……能除毁痛,皆自然之理也"。"肝病用大嘘三十遍,细嘘十遍,自然去肝家虚热,亦除四肢壮热、眼暗、一切烦热等。数数嘘之,绵绵相次不绝为妙。病差,止。过度则损"。

'The vibration of the *Xu* sound helps to alleviate liver problems. The *Xu* sound can soothe liver qi ... relieve pain in the rib-side area.' '30 times of loud *Xu* sound coupled with 10 times of low *Xu* sound clear heat in the liver and alleviate fever in four limbs, blurred vision and vexation. Repeat the sound uninterruptedly and stop when your health condition is improved. Excessive vibration of the sound may harm your body'.

2. 呵的应用
2. The *He* sound

"心之有疾,当用呵,呵者,心之气……呵能静其心,和其神。所以人之昏乱者多呵,盖天然之气也。故心病当用呵泻之也"。"以鼻微长引气,以口呵之,皆调气如上,勿令自耳闻之,然后呵之。心有病用大呵三十遍、细呵十遍,去心家劳热、一切烦闷。

疾差止，过度损"。

'The vibration of the *He* sound helps to alleviate heart problems. The *Xu* sound can calm and clear the heart-mind.' 'Inhale with the nose and exhale with the *He* sound from the mouth silently. 30 times of loud *He* sound coupled with 10 times of low *He* sound can clear heat in the heart and alleviate heat sensation and vexation. Stop when your health condition is improved. Excessive vibration of the sound may harm your body'.

3. 呼的应用
3. The *Hu* sound

"脾之有疾，当用呼，呼者，脾之气……能抽脾之疾，故人中热者，则呼以驱其弊也"。"脾病，用大呼三十遍，细呼十遍，能去脾家一切冷气，发热霍乱，宿食不消，偏风麻痹，腹内结块，数数呼之，相次勿绝，疾退则止，过度则损"。

'The vibration of the *Hu* sound helps to alleviate spleen problems. The *Hu* sound can regulate spleen qi and clear heat in the spleen and stomach'. '30 times of loud *Hu* sound coupled with 10 times of low *Hu* sound warm the spleen and alleviate fever, cholera, poor digestion, hemiplegia and abdominal masses. Repeat the sound uninterruptedly and stop when your health condition is improved. Excessive vibration of the sound may harm your body'.

4. 呬的应用
4. The *Hei* sound

"肺之有疾，当用呬。呬者，肺之气也……能抽肺之疾，所以人之有怨气填塞胸臆者，则长呬而泻之，盖自然之理也"。"以鼻微长引气，以口呬之，勿令耳闻。皆先调气令和，然后呬之。肺有病，用大呬三十遍，细呬十遍，去劳热上气，咳嗽，皮肤疮疡，四肢劳烦，鼻塞，胸背疼痛。依法呬疾，差止，过度则损"。

'The vibration of the *Si* (*Hei*) sound helps to alleviate lung problems. The *Si* (*Hei*) sound can regulate lung qi and alleviate tightness or oppression in the chest'. 'Inhale with the nose and exhale with the *Si* (*Hei*) sound from the mouth silently. 30 times of loud *Si* (*Hei*) sound coupled with 10 times of low *Si* (*Hei*) sound reduce fever, alleviate cough, skin sores or ulcers, weakness of the four limbs, nasal obstruction, chest and back pain. Stop when your health condition is improved. Excessive vibration of the sound may harm your body'.

5. 吹的应用
5. The *Chui* sound

"肾之有疾，当用吹，吹者，肾之气……能抽肾之疾，故人有积气冲臆者，则强吹也，肾气沉滞，重吹则渐通也"。"肾病用大吹三十遍，细吹十遍，能去肾家一切冷腰疼、膝冷、腰脚沉重，久立不得，阳道衰弱。耳中虫鸣，及口中有疮，是肾家诸疾，诸烦热悉皆去之。数数吹之，相次勿绝，疾差则止，过度则损"。

'The vibration of the *Chui* sound helps to alleviate kidney problems. The *Chui* sound can supplement kidney qi'. '30 times of loud *Chui* sound coupled with 10 times of low *Chui* sound alleviate low back pain, a cold sensation in the knee joints, heaviness of the low back and leg, inability to stand for long period of time, tinnitus, mouth ulceration and feverish sensation. Repeat the sound uninterruptedly and stop when your health condition is improved. Excessive vibration of the sound may harm your body'.

6. 嘻的应用
6. The *Xi* sound

"治胆用嘻,嘻为补,吸为泻","以鼻渐长引气,以口嘻之,去胆家病,并阴脏除一切冷,阴汗,盗汗,面无颜色,小肠胀满,口下冷痛,口干舌涩,数嘻之,疾乃愈"。

'The vibration of the *Xi* sound helps to alleviate gallbladder problems. "Inhaling with the nose and exhaling with the *Xi* sound from the mouth can stop cold or night sweats, a pale complexion, intestinal fullness and distension, and a dry mouth and tongue'.

在具体应用中,可以通过五行的相生相克理论在治疗上加以运用,如金元医学四大家之一的刘完素,在他所撰的《素问玄机原病式》一书中述:"脏腑之六气,实则行其本化之字泻之,衰则行其胜己之字泻之。"

In terms of treatment, mutual promotion and inhibition among the five elements can be applied to actual practice. For example, Liu Wan-su[1] stated in his *Su Wen Xuan Ji Yuan Bing Shuo* (Explanation of Mysterious Pathogeneses and Etiologies Based on the 'Basic Questions'), 'For excessive syndrome of the zang-fu, reduce with the sound for the mutually promoted organ; and for deficient syndrome of the zang-fu organs, reduce with the sound for the mutually inhibited organ'.

---

1. Liu Wansu (aka Liu Hejian, 1120–1200): One of the four great masters of the Jin-Yuan era and representative of the Cold and Cooling School.

而在养生方面，六字诀显示出了有病治病、无病养生的效果。明代太医院的龚廷贤在他著的《寿世保元》中说："五脏六腑之气，因五味熏灼不知，又六欲七情，积久生病，内伤脏腑，外攻九窍……其法以呼字而自泻去脏腑之毒气，以吸气而自采天地之清气补气。当日小验，旬日大验，年后百病不生，延年益寿。卫生之宝，非人勿传。"

In addition to disease treatment, the six healing sounds are helpful to disease prevention. Gong Tingxian (1522–1619) stated in his *Shou Shi Bao Yuan* (*Prolonging Life and Preserving the Origin*), 'Over time, five flavors, seven emotions and six sensory pleasures may cause qi disorder of the five-zang and six-fu organs ... one needs to inhale clean qi from the nature to supplement qi and exhale to remove turbid qi from the zang-fu organs. One can feel good after practice for even one day, better after 10 days and stay away from any diseases after 1 year'.

现 代 应 用

Modern application

六字诀的医疗和养生效果在现代的实践应用中都得到了验证，虽然目前的几个版本在发声和动作不尽相同，但在应用功效上都表现出相应的作用。我们按照六字的对应应用加以总结。

The role of six healing sounds in health care and cultivation has been widely recognized. Despite differences in method and vibration of the sounds, current versions or styles share similar functions. The indications of each sound are summarized as follows:

1. 嘘

1. The *Xu* sound (for liver qi)

肝气诀：适用于肝炎、肝火旺、肝肿大、胸肋胀闷、食欲不振、青光眼、两目干涩、眼中赤色兼多泪、高血压、低血压、头目眩晕等病症。

Indications: Hepatitis, hyperactivity of liver fire, hepatomegaly, distension and tightness in the chest and rib-side area, a poor appetite, glaucoma, dry eyes, red eyes or lacrimation, hypertension, hypotension, dizziness and blurred vision.

2. 呵

2. The *He* sound (for heart qi)

心气诀：适用于心脏病、心悸、心绞痛、心神烦躁、失眠、健忘、盗汗、口舌糜烂、生疮、舌强语言謇及热痛等病症。

Indications: Heart diseases, palpitations, angina pectoris, restlessness, insomnia, poor memory, night sweats, mouth or tongue ulceration, tongue stiffness, fever and pain.

3. 呼

3. The *Hu* sound (for spleen qi)

脾气诀：适用于肠胃炎、胃胀、腹泻、四肢疲乏、食欲不振、痰湿热生、吐水、肌肉萎缩、皮肤水肿等病症。

Indications: Gastroenteritis, stomach distension, abdominal

diarrhea, weakness of the four limbs, a poor appetite, phlegm-damp and heat, vomiting of watery fluid, muscular atrophy and edema.

4. 呬
4. The *Hei* sound (for lung qi)

肺气诀: 适用于气管炎、咳嗽、痰涎、胸膈烦躁、喉舌干等病症。

Indications: Tracheitis/bronchitis, cough, profuse phlegm, chest and diaphragm discomfort and a dry tongue or throat.

5. 吹
5. The *Chui* sound (for kidney qi)

肾气诀: 适用于腰膝酸软、耳鸣、盗汗遗精、阳痿、早泄、肾结石、子宫虚寒、黑瘦等病症。

Indications: Soreness and weakness in the low back and knee joints, tinnitus, night sweats, nocturnal emissions, premature ejaculation, kidney stones, deficiency and cold in the uterus and a dark-gray complexion with weight loss.

6. 嘻
6. The *Xi* sound (for Sanjiao qi)

三焦诀: 适用于三焦不畅通而引起的眩晕、耳鸣、喉痛、胸腹胀闷、小便不利等疾患。

Indications: Vertigo, tinnitus, sore throat, distension and tightness in the chest and abdomen and dysuria.

总而言之，古音六字诀可以调整虚实寒热，调理气机，畅通经络，调节脏腑功能，故在治疗和养生的应用中有着广泛的应用。

In summary, the six healing sounds are extensively used in treatment and health cultivation because they can help to regulate deficiency, excess, cold, heat and qi activity, unblock meridians, and harmonize functions of the zang-fu organs.

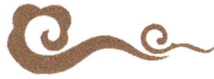

古 音 六 字 诀　•　*Gu Yin Liu Zi Jue* (Six Healing Sounds)

The Meridian Charts

经络图

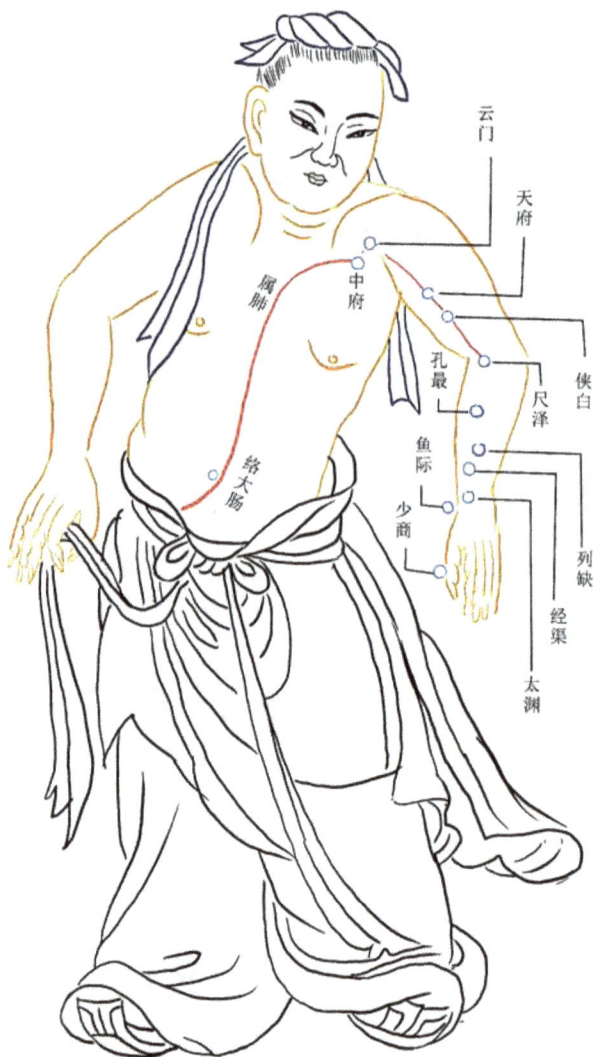

云门
天府
中府
属肺
侠白
孔最
尺泽
鱼际
络大肠
列缺
少商
经渠
太渊

手太阴肺经

Lung Meridian of Hand-Taiyin

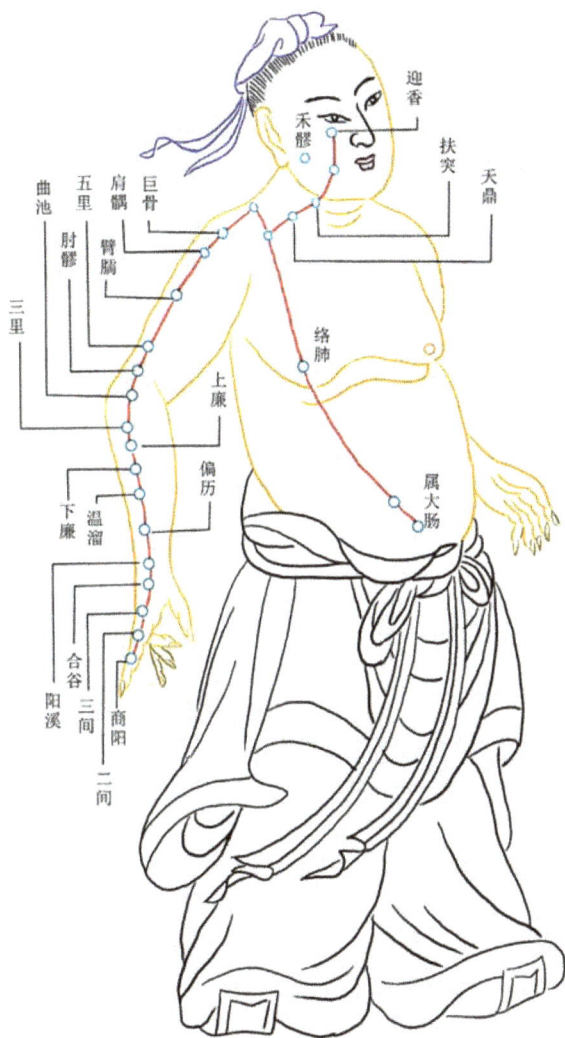

迎香
扶突
天鼎
禾髎
巨骨
肩髃
曲池
五里
臂臑
肘髎
三里
络肺
上廉
偏历
温溜
下廉
合谷
阳溪
三间
商阳
二间
属大肠

手阳明大肠经

Large Intestine Meridian of Hand-Yangming

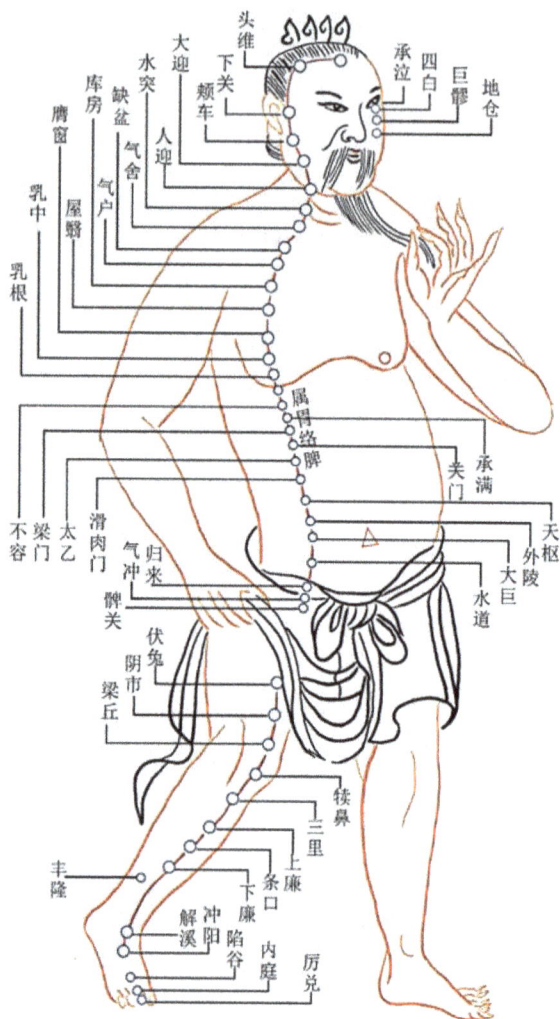

头维　下关　颊车　承泣　四白　巨髎　地仓
大迎　水突　人迎　缺盆　气舍　气户
库房　膺窗　屋翳　乳中　乳根　气冲
属胃络脾　关门　承满　天枢　外陵　大巨　水道
滑肉门　太乙　梁门　不容　归来　髀关　伏兔　阴市　梁丘
犊鼻　三里　上廉　条口　下廉　冲阳　陷谷　内庭　厉兑
丰隆　解溪

足阳明胃经

Stomach Meridian of Foot-Yangming

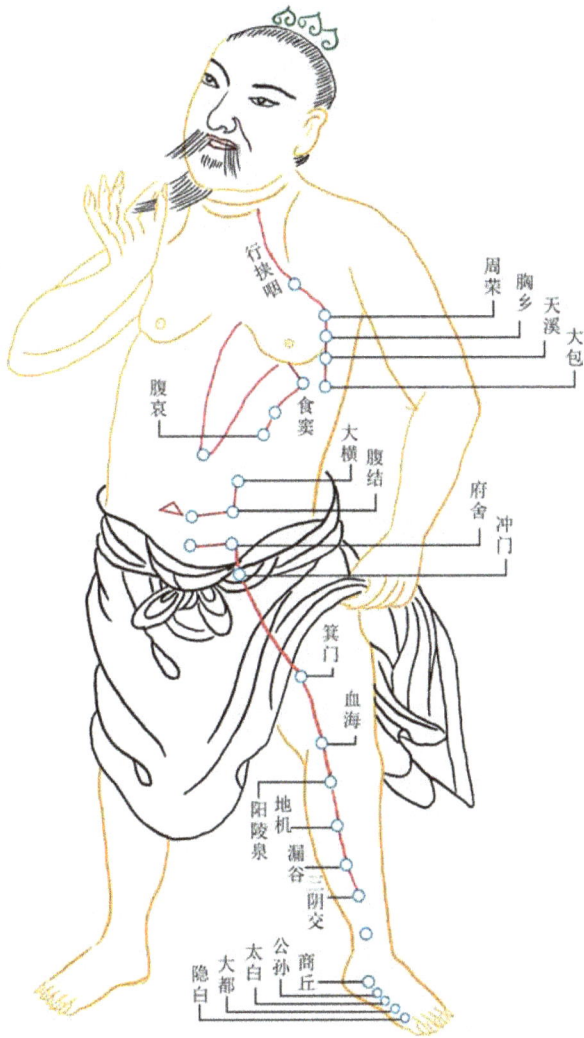

足太阴脾经

Spleen Meridian of Foot-Taiyin

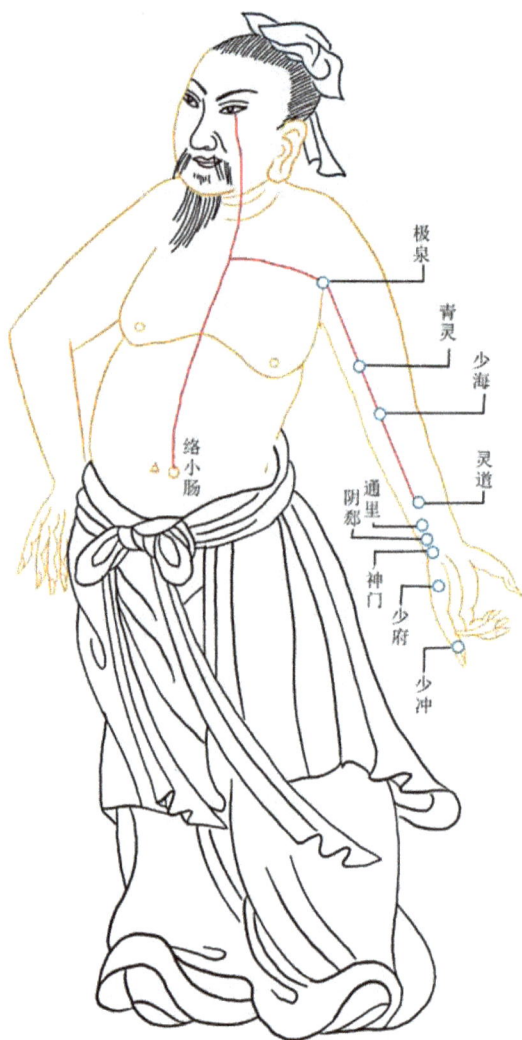

极泉

青灵

少海

灵道

通里
阴郄

神门

少府

少冲

络
小肠

手少阴心经

Heart Meridian of Hand-Shaoyin

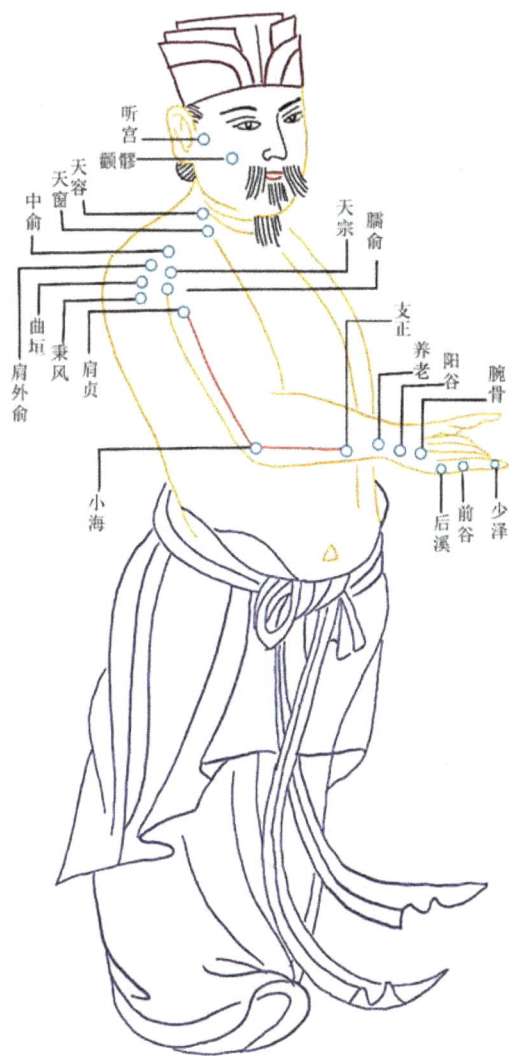

听宫
颧髎
天容
天窗
中俞
曲垣
秉风
肩贞
肩外俞
小海
天宗
膈俞
支正
养老
阳谷
腕骨
后溪
前谷
少泽

手太阳小肠经

Small Intestine Meridian of Hand-Taiyang

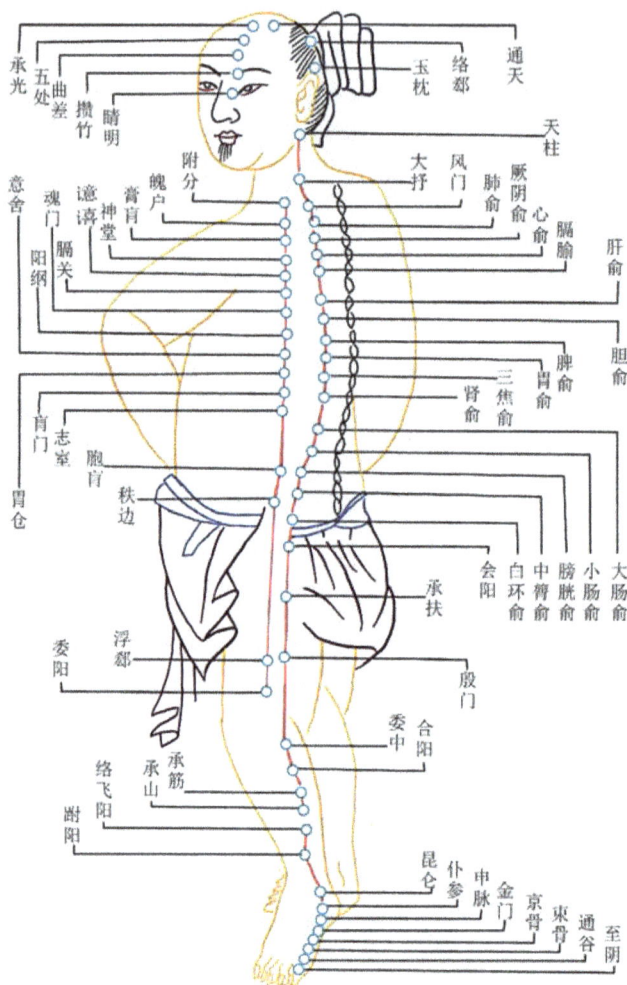

足太阳膀胱经

Bladder Meridian of Foot-Taiyang

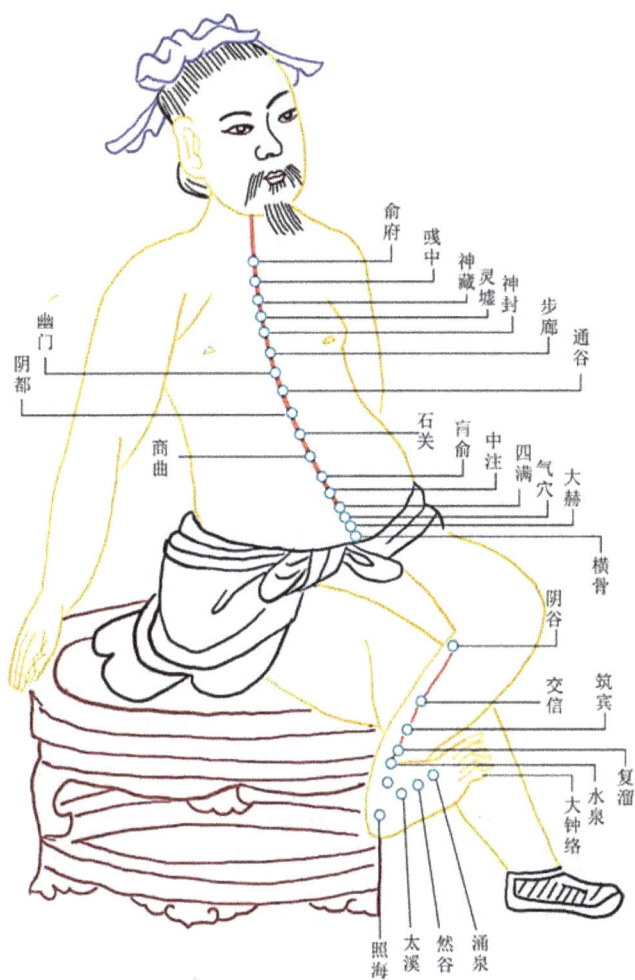

足少阴肾经

Kidney Meridian of Foot-Shaoyin

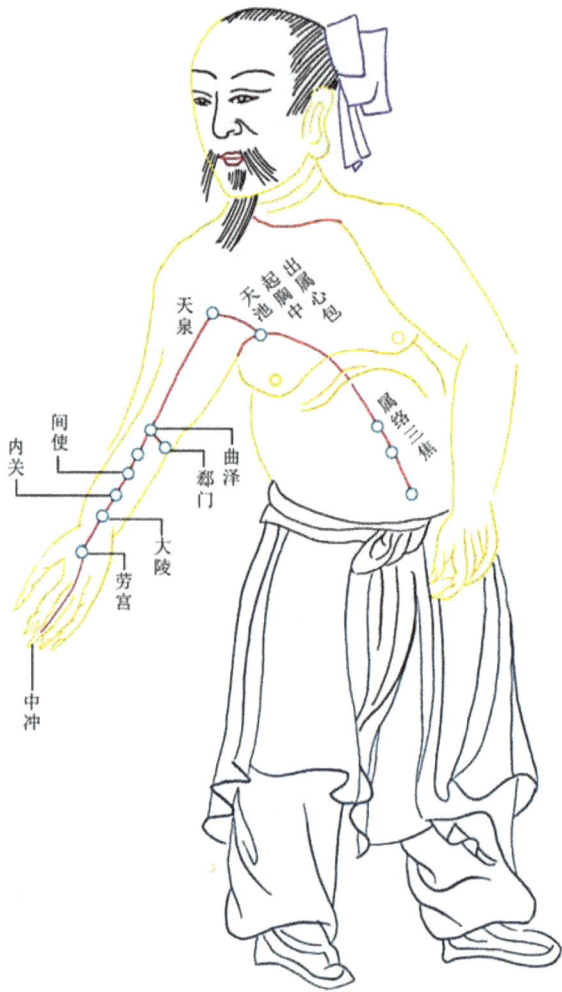

天池
起膈中
出属心包
天泉
属络三焦
间使
内关
曲泽
郄门
大陵
劳宫
中冲

手厥阴心包经

Pericardium Meridian of Hand-Jueyin

手少阳三焦经

Triple Energizer Meridian of Hand-Shaoyang

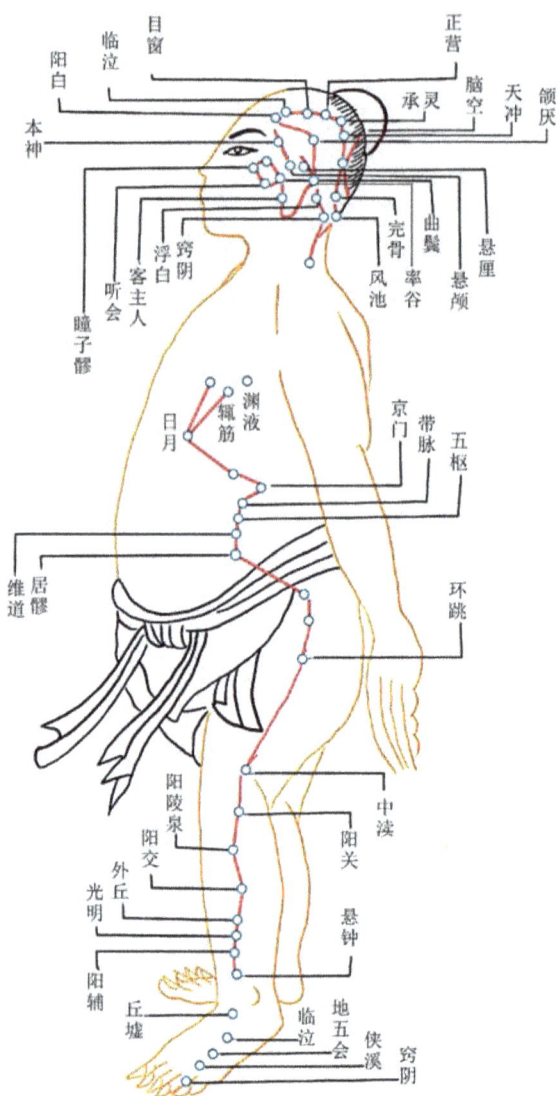

足少阳胆经

Gallbladder Meridian of Foot-Shaoyang

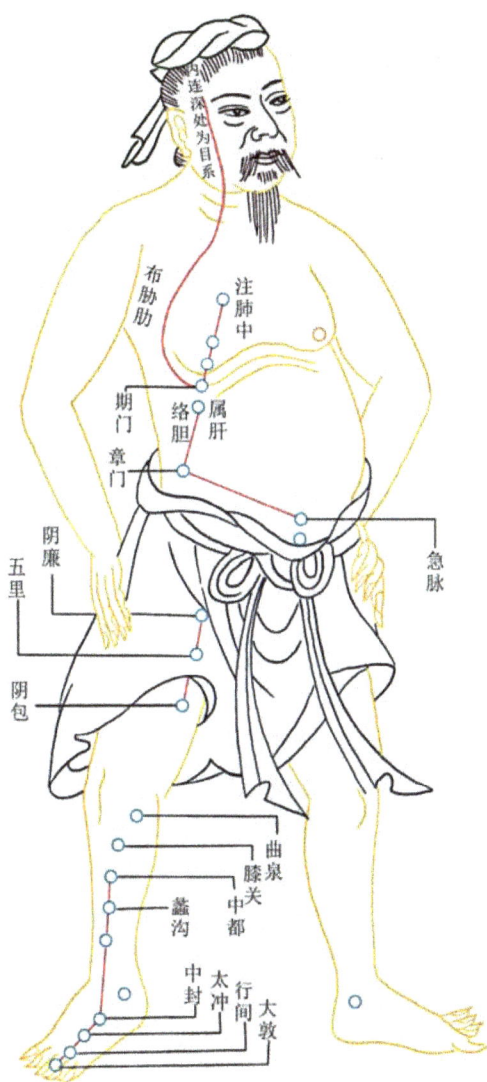

足厥阴肝经

Liver Meridian of Foot-Jueyin

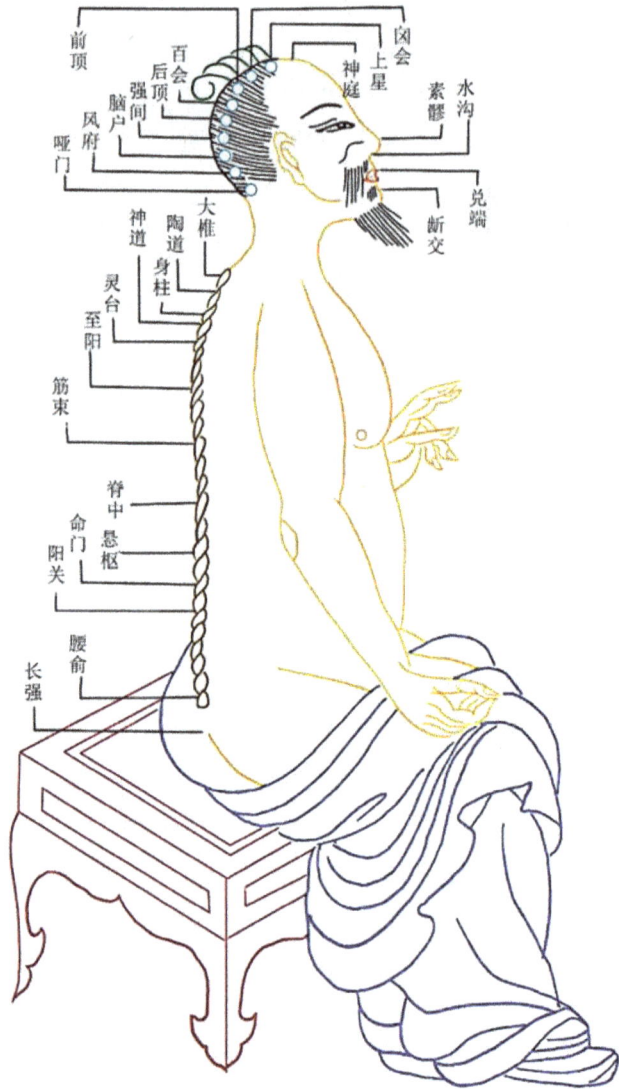

前顶
百会
后顶
强间
脑户
风府
哑门
囟会
上星
神庭
素髎
水沟
兑端
龂交
大椎
陶道
身柱
神道
灵台
至阳
筋束
脊中
悬枢
命门
阳关
腰俞
长强

督脉

Governor Vessel (Du)

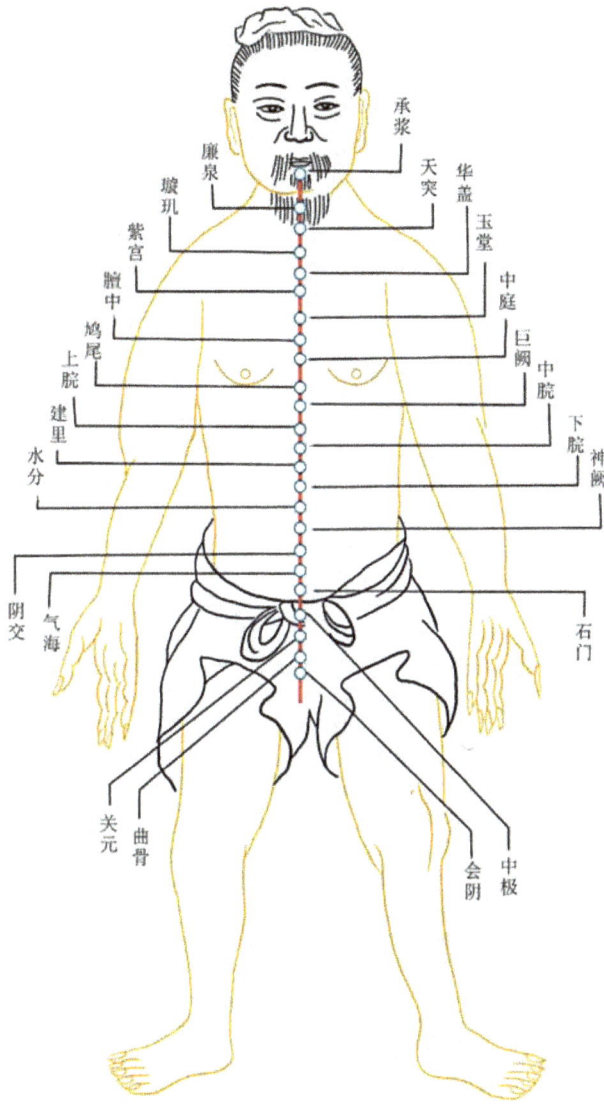

承浆
廉泉
璇玑
紫宫
膻中
鸠尾
上脘
建里
水分
阴交
气海
关元
曲骨
会阴
中极
石门
神阙
下脘
中脘
巨阙
中庭
玉堂
华盖
天突

任脉

Conception Vessel (Ren)

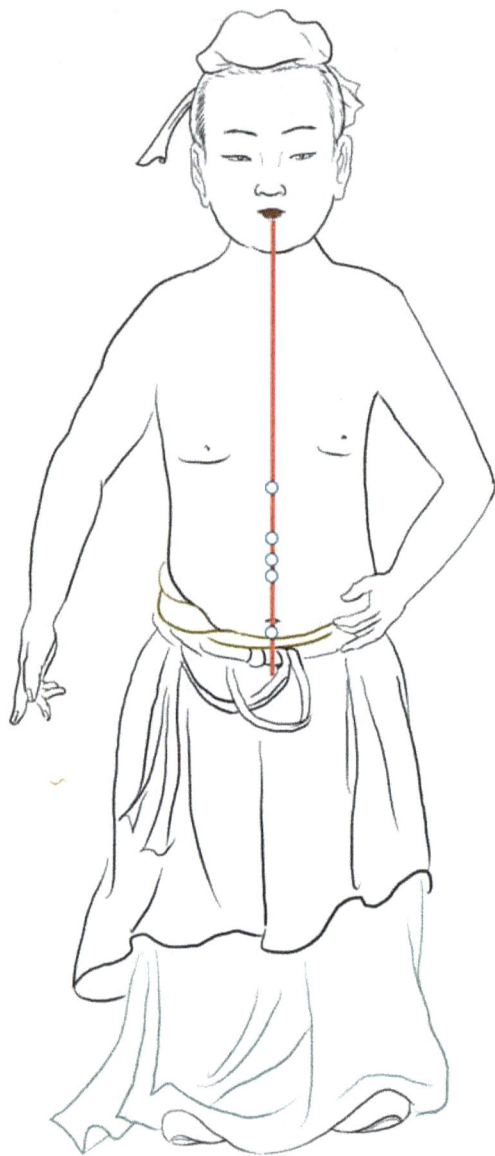

冲脉

Thoroughfare Vessel (Chong)

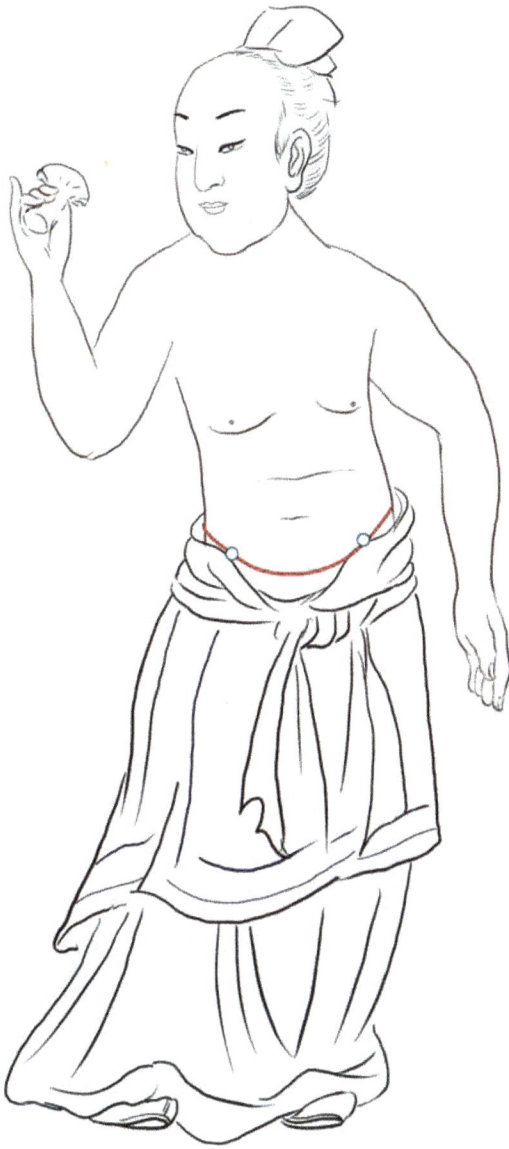

带脉

Belt Vessel (Dai)

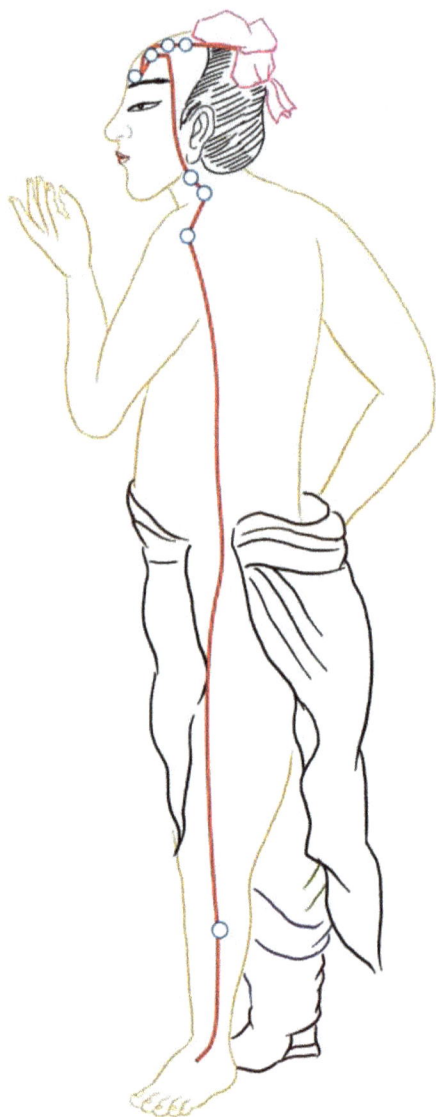

阳维脉

Yang Link Vessel (Yang Wei)

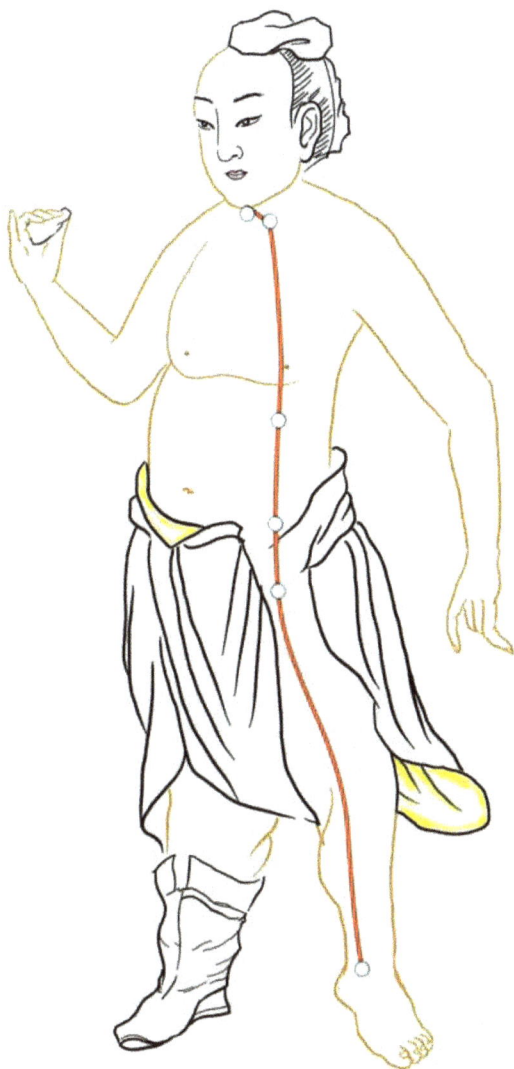

阴维脉

Yin Link Vessel (Yin Wei)

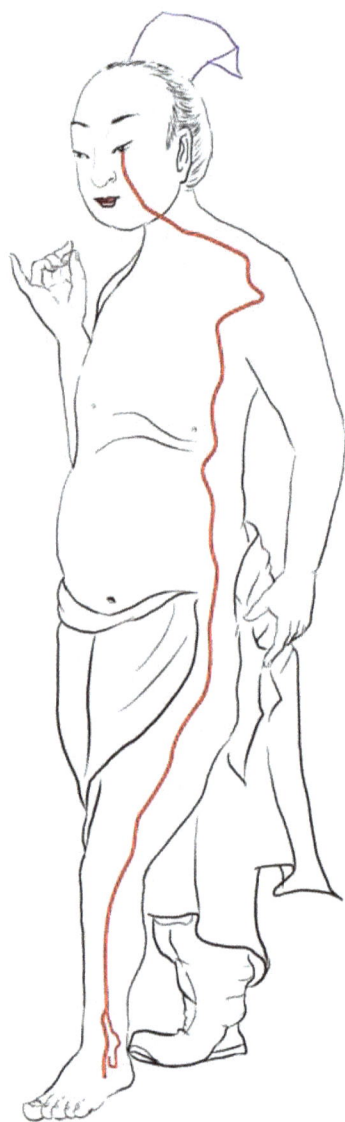

阳蹻脉

Yang Heel Vessel (Yang Qiao)

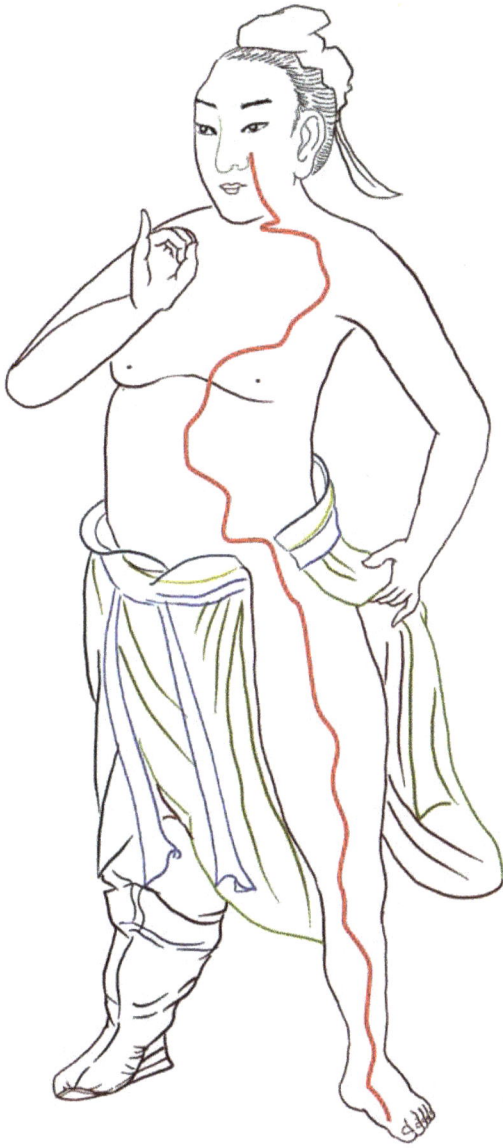

阴蹻脉

Yin Heel Vessel (Yin Qiao)